# The Laminitis Bible

# The Laminitis Bible

*42 Years Preventing Founder in Over 1,200 Real Cases*

By Dr. David Frederick

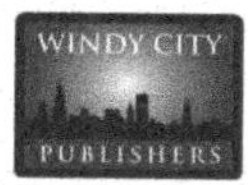

The Laminitis Bible



Windy City Publishers
www.windycitypublishers.com

Published in the United States of America

ISBN#:
978-1-953294-22-7

Library of Congress Control Number:
2021922736

Windy City Publishers
Chicago

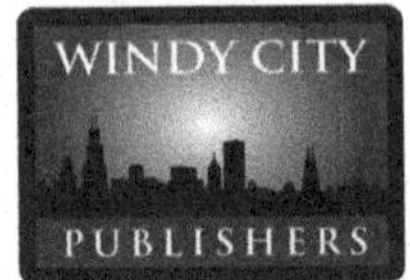

# Contents

# Acknowledgments

I WROTE THE MORE THAN 50 laminitis stories in this book on a series of four different computers over about 35 years. I might have written the first couple on an electric typewriter. I have had a series of editors try to help me bring them together into a book. All offered constructive criticism. Too often their efforts to smooth out my grammar, or rough punctuation, changed what I was trying to say. I have always insisted on accuracy being far more important to me than style. I have left in a few repetitions because repetition is the way I learn. These are real cases, and I have written them as I saw them. Two people seeing the same thing can often describe it differently, but this is what I saw in each case.

After the individual cases were completed, my final three editors, Dr. David Ahrenholz, Sandy Remmers, and Karla Kreklow, went through the entire book several times. I will be forever grateful for their knowledge, talent, focus, and determination to finally get this book printed. All three are very successful horse owners. They absolutely represent my target audience. It is my hope that the entire horse owning public will become as comfortable with the difference between laminitis and founder as they have become. This requires understanding the difference between Vasocompression and Vasoconstriction. Knowing the difference will be life or death for your horse until the professors get it right.

I was the only student in my graduating class in 1974 to go straight into his own private solo vet practice. I could not have done this without some outstanding mentors to help me whenever I saw something for the first time. Dr. Walt Dalitsch graduated 11 years before me and was the most frequent help my entire career. When I got in trouble with a colic, a difficult foaling, or a toxicity I had never seen before, I called Dr. Dalitsch. He has been a great friend for over 44 years and celebrated his 55th year in practice in 2018! We have covered for each other's short vacations since I graduated. Dr. Dalitsch was the first to teach me how to treat laminitis, and I have never had to change his anti-inflammatory approach.

I had several outstanding professors in vet school, whom I am sure had no idea what I might remember from their lectures, but I remember like it was yesterday. Doctors Erv Small said, "You MUST examine the animal," Harry Hardenbrook said, "There is no way you can describe what you saw on a horse's leg to me. I MUST see the horse," and Don Lindgard said, "Failure to do a rectal exam on a colic is malpractice." They, of course, shared much longer stories to drive home their points, but I got those messages from them.

Two more long-term mentors were Dr. Paul Smith, a brilliant state vet at the harness tracks whom I pestered with questions for over 20 years. He frequently said to me, "Wait 'til you've killed a few, son," as his way of putting my silly questions into perspective. I've tried very hard to never kill a horse that did not need to be killed. The late Dr. Tom Phillips, who owned the Illinois Equine Clinic, was, by far, the most valuable emergency help for me when I was in serious trouble with a colic, or any disease or lameness I could not figure out. I sent a couple hundred horses to his clinic over 25 years (until his retirement), but I never had to send him a horse with laminitis. He was incredibly patient with my forever education on all the other diseases. I never graduated from his classes. *Tuesdays with Morrie* could have been written about Dr. Phillips.

The Illinois Racing Board gave me a scholarship which enabled me to ride along a week each with 10 different vets before my last year of vet school. This let me watch Doctors Alex Harthill, Ken Walker, Ron "Swede" Jensen, Joe Foerner, Tom White, Walt Dalitsch, and others in action. A week at Castleton Farm let me see how things were done in Lexington. Other vets unintentionally showed me what does not work so well.

At least 30 hours of Continuing Education is required every two years for license renewal, so I have attended many vet conventions around the country and heard the national experts lecture for years. Some are much better than others. A few of my favorites are/were Doctors Nat White, Jim Moore, Bill Donawick, DeWitt Owen, Robert Copeland, Sue Dyson, Tracy Turner, Amber LaBelle, Bill Moyer, Susan White, Eleanor Green, Bill Stone and Chris Pollitt.

There have been literally hundreds of research articles published in rigid, peer reviewed veterinary journals examining different aspects of laminitis the past 45 years. I may have read and tried to understand at least half of the scientific articles in the laminitis literature. The vast majority of them are fully compatible with my vasocompression approach. None of them have been able to prove the vasoconstriction theory still favored by the majority of the researchers. Some of the most significant studies, which I believe support vasocompression were published by Doctors Jim Coffman, David Hood, Harold Garner, Jim Moore, Doug Allen, Robert Bowker, and of course Chris Pollitt, among many others.

I have met, written to, and tried to discuss my laminitis opinions with many of these prominent laminitis researchers and lecturers, but they are a closed group which, as a general rule, has little time or interest in looking at or listening to my 42 years of over 1,200 "anecdotes." None have ever accepted my invitations to come see many of my survivors of really severe laminitis or examine my records which these case reports are based on, or speak with the owners, who in most cases have reviewed and approved their horse's case reports. New research studies seem far more important to the Laminitis Research Industry than preventing foundered horses.

Deserving the biggest thanks for teaching me so much about such an important subject have been my patients and their wonderful owners who have trusted my advice and help for so many years. The more than 50 stories in this book have been selected for their teaching value. They represent the full spectrum of the disease, but the failures are way overrepresented, because we can learn so much more from our failures than our successes. The vast majority of the cures are very short stories, most requiring only one or two visits. But every case is a little different.

You, the responsible horse owner, will have to read this book yourself, and buy another for your vet as a Christmas present. Discuss a specific case from the book with him before you pay your next bill. Only by forcing the vets to talk about it will they overcome what they were taught in school—that laminitis is a mysterious disease which needs more research. You must be your horse's strongest advocate to see that he gets the attention and correct care he deserves.

FAMILY NOTE:

With all due respect to the "final three editors,
Dr. David Ahrenholz, Sandy Remmers, and Karla Krecklow"
(noted on page xi in paragraph 2),
we must tell you that Dr. Frederick passed away before his book
was moved to the publisher selected by Dr. Frederick,
who unfortunately had just closed their doors.

At that time, Dr. Frederick's wife and children asked Dr. Frederick's
brother Tom of Highlands Ranch, Colorado, to find a new publisher,
who had new formatting requirements, and bring the book to the
marketplace. That was no easy task given the onset of COVID restrictions
that impacted everyone's "normal."

Dr. Frederick's wife Julie still lives on their newly built retirement
horse property outside Landrum, South Carolina.

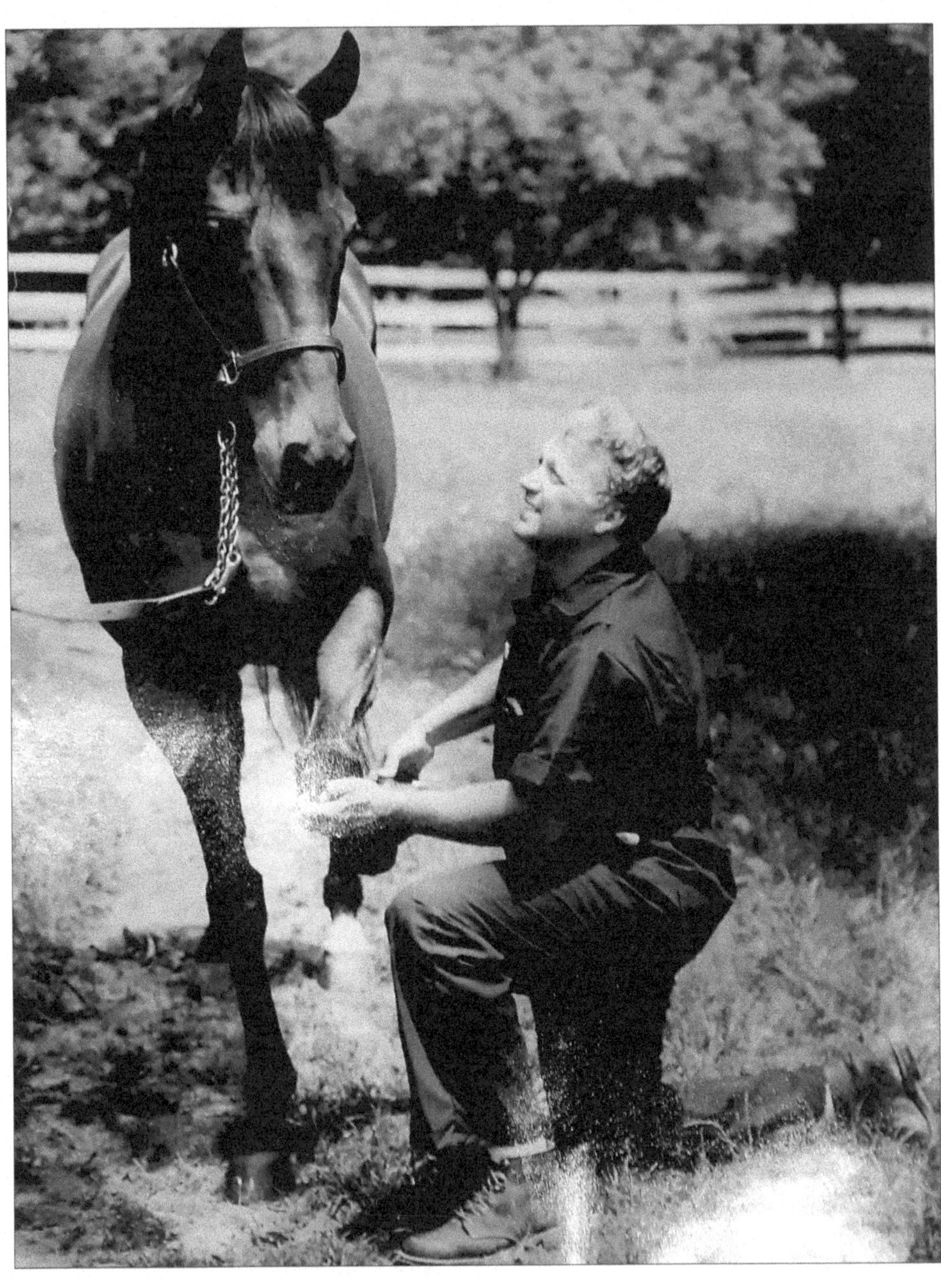

# Introduction

THE PURPOSE OF THIS BOOK is to summarize what I have learned in 42 years of private equine practice treating acute laminitis. The goal is not to criticize any horse owner, veterinarian, or farrier, but to illustrate the all too easy errors in diagnosis and treatment of this medical emergency in horses. Each horse's presentation can be dramatic or subtle, but early diagnosis, elimination of the triggering event, and a consistent, logical approach to treatment are the best way to prevent crippling founder in our horses. Your vet should be consulted at the first signs of lameness.

For the past 30 years, I have felt like David shooting pebbles with my sling shot at the Laminitis Research Industry. I have been telling everyone who I think can make a difference, that Acute Laminitis is the easiest disease I get to treat (1,2). Since my first year of Veterinary School, I have always understood it better than any other disease. If I am called at the first sign of lameness, or even before lameness, if the horse gets into the grain barrel, it has always been very simple for me to treat and prevent founder.

I have euthanized 26 horses because of uncontrollable founder pain, but every one of them was due to human error—never the "mysterious nature of the disease" which needed more research to understand. Millions of dollars of research already supports my view that inflammation and edema cause vasocompression and laminitis. Unfortunately, many researchers and professors continue to try to make the research fit vasoconstriction theories. They have been failing for 40 years.

The more than 50 case histories in this book are each just an "anecdote" individually, but they were chosen for their teaching value. We learn much more from our failures than from our successes, so the failures are way over-represented in these case histories.

It is my hope that all people who love and care for horses will read a chapter of this book every morning or night much like people who love God read a verse of the Bible every day. There are many different presentations of Acute Laminitis. I have seen more than a thousand over the past 42 years. Unlike founder, Acute Laminitis is very treatable if recognized and treated properly. The conscientious horseman must read these unique case histories, learn to identify and remove the inciting causes, and recognize the disease early so that it is treated properly from day one.

# Peer Pressure and Peer Review

*Grade school, high school, vet school...*
*unions, political parties, and professionals*

I SKATED THROUGH GRADE SCHOOL and high school bouncing between the athletes and top students, never feeling any peer pressure to join either group to the exclusion of the other. Sports were my big interest. My best athletic success was on the track, where I set a record in the half mile run that was not broken for many decades. Of course, I had no idea then that I would wander into the world of horses racing around a track, resulting in the care of four legged athletes becoming my life's work. In the classroom, math was very easy for me. I often found my own ways to solve algebra and geometry problems when I hadn't paid enough attention to remember the formulas the teacher had shown us the day before. Throughout my life I have never been shy about challenging authority (starting with teachers and coaches) when I saw things differently.

However, vet school at the University of Illinois was not so easy—very little math, and far too much chemistry. It was where I was really indoctrinated with the union mentality. "Ethics" was drummed into us. I was told, "Never criticize another veterinarian." "You weren't there." "You have no idea why one animal responds positively, and another with exactly the same symptoms and treatments responds negatively." "You cannot comment on a case you were not personally involved with." "Never guarantee success." "Sometimes an animal will recover in spite of your screw ups." "Never assume anything you did was the reason an animal got well." "Do not brag about saving 10 in a row, because the next 10 might die, and then you will have to take the blame, if you want the credit for the survivors."

Yes, our animals are all unique individuals, and no two sets of circumstances are exactly alike in living organisms, but we do have to learn from our mistakes.

That is why we "practice." Whether it is sports, music, math, medicine, or flying an airplane, we all must practice if we want to improve. A 90-year-old violin master was asked why he still practiced four hours every day. He answered simply, "Because I think I notice some improvement when I practice."

The supposed gold standard for veterinary researchers is the "Double Blind" clinical trial. This involves randomly splitting a group in half and giving a specific treatment to half the patients and a placebo treatment to the other half. Neither the patients, nor the researcher knows which have received the treatment being tested. The results are assessed by another researcher who had nothing to do with the treatment. Only after the results are recorded is the treated group identified for tabulation. A result showing 15 of 20 treated improved versus 9 of 20 untreated improving is considered "scientific evidence" and readily publishable in "peer-reviewed" scientific journals, to show the tested drug is better than nothing. The FDA might then approve the new drug, or they might ask for "Open Label" clinical trials as the next step. These unblinded clinical trials do not require a control or untreated group, but investigator bias could influence the results.

Open Label clinical trials involve much greater numbers than double blind trials. I have tested my personal approach to laminitis since 1974, by following my clinical outcomes. For the first 15 years, I tracked all my laminitis failures. Since then, I have recorded all my laminitis cases regardless of their outcomes.

Laminitis treatments can likely never be proven with double blind trials. There are simply too many variables that dictate how much treatment is necessary. The disease has two very different stages, which make it vital to treat early for consistent results. As early as 1905, Dennis Magner wrote in *Magner's Standard Horse and Stock Book* (3), "Every case of acute laminitis is curable if treated properly, which is not at all difficult...but, if not treated promptly, the chronic stage is not curable...and (the horse) is practically ruined."

Since the day I graduated, laminitis has been the easiest disease for me to diagnosis and treat successfully. I did make a few mistakes which cost horses their lives, and I tell their stories in this book along with many others where the owners, trainers, or other vets made errors leading to death. Some vets believe my method may work for the mild laminitis cases, but that other cases are so advanced that nothing can save them. Those were much more rare in my practice because the vast majority were correctly treated at the beginning of the disease because the owner or responsible caregiver called me early in the disease state. I have included a fair number that were extremely severe on day one or two but fully recovered and returned to prior use. Some others were cured of laminitis while they were dying of colic, peritonitis, and kidney failure. Each of the case histories was chosen for its teaching value. We all can learn far more from our mistakes than from our successes.

I could never finish this book until I was forced to retire at age seventy due to Pulmonary Fibrosis. I loved my work, and there was always something new to learn. These stories were written over a forty-year time frame, on four different computers and achieving a printable form has been a challenge for my editors. Sadly, some very good stories written years ago were lost. Just a few, I retold from memory rather than written clinical records.

I have always tried to be as accurate as possible while trying to honor individual privacy. A person's perception is reality to them. This book is the way I saw these events happen.

Unless your horse is in a crisis, do not try to read this book in a few days or a week. The cases will all run together, and you will not learn nearly as much. It is best to read a case a day, or even a case a week. Or buy a second book for your vet or trainer and ask them to discuss one or more of these reports. A handful of case illustrations are just anecdotes which prove nothing, but at some point, when the same approach consistently works over a 42-year period, those with an open mind will realize that early treatment of the inflammation is far better than delayed symptomatic treatment.

Everyone learns some things by trial and error. One of my professors said if there are a dozen different treatments for a disease, it's because none of them work consistently. That was never the case for me with laminitis. Too many vets use trial and error their entire career, treating laminitis with inconsistent results.

# Acute Laminitis versus Founder

## *Definitions and Outcomes*

THIS BOOK IS A COMPENDIUM of 40 plus years of my clinical experience treating acute laminitis in horses and ponies. It includes more than 50 case histories, some of which are spectacular failures, but included for illustrative purposes. Acute laminitis is extremely common and has a variety of triggering events that we shall discuss shortly. Far too many owners and others confuse the term "laminitis" with "founder."

**Acute laminitis is an inflammation within the hoof**, characterized by gradual or sudden onset of lameness in horses, frequently affecting the forelegs before the hind legs. In 1948, Dr. Obel (4) rated the severity of lameness on a scale from I to IV.

### GRADE I

Horses shift weight from one foot to the other or repeatedly lift feet. Lameness is not evident at a walk, but at the trot horses have a shortened stride.

### GRADE II

Horses move willingly at a walk and trot but with a noticeably shortened stride. A foot can be lifted off the ground without difficulty.

### GRADE III

Horses move reluctantly, and resist attempts to lift affected or contralateral feet.

## GRADE IV

Horses express marked reluctance or absolute refusal to move. Founder is a horseman's term for chronic lameness from unrecognized or inadequately treated acute laminitis. With chronic laminitis there is progressive detachment of the hoof from the coffin bone. Chronic or recurrent lameness limits the horse's movements and is often associated with a rocking behavior as the horse alternates unloading each painful hoof. In the most severe cases the coffin bone rotates or sinks downward within the hoof, possibly even penetrating through the sole.

Some of our most famous racehorses including Secretariat, Nihilator (with more than $3 million pacing winnings), Evening Snow (World Record quarter mile), Hall of Famer Bold 'N Determined, and Barbaro have died of "incurable" laminitis despite the finest and most up-to-date veterinary and farrier care available.

Dr. Ric Redden of the International Equine Podiatry Center, a master at saving desperate cases, has twice told American Association of Equine Practitioners members (5,6) that 20 percent of all laminitis cases become complicated "regardless of therapy" and 80 percent remain non-complicated "with or without treatment."

That's quite different from Magner's quote, "Every case of acute laminitis is curable if treated properly, which is not at all difficult...but, if not treated promptly, the chronic stage is not curable...and (the horse) is practically ruined," (3) which, in my experience, has shown to be true.

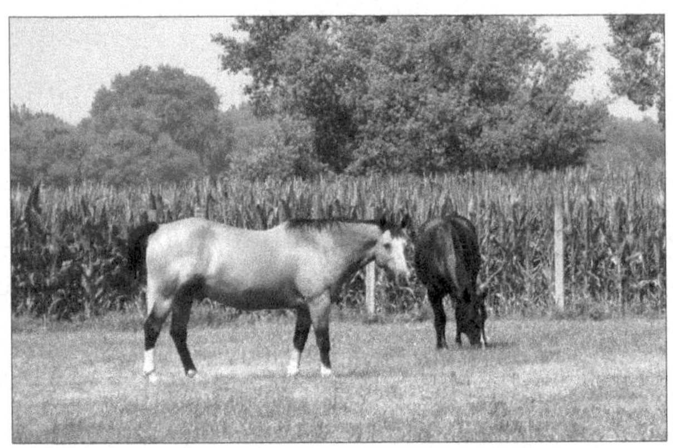

*Neither of these very fat horses developed Laminitis in 15 years on this pasture.*

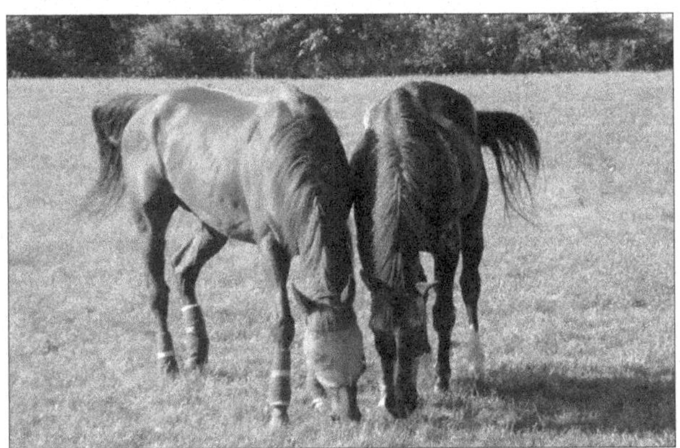

*Both of these thin horses repeatedly developed Mild Acute Laminitis on this pasture.*

# Multiple Causes of Acute Laminitis

A NUMBER OF APPARENTLY UNRELATED conditions can trigger acute laminitis. Most common is a change in diet with increased consumption of simple carbohydrates (sugars). This can occur during lush pasture growth when plants rapidly produce these sugars, also called non-structural carbohydrates (NSCs), in response to good growing conditions such as the springtime. These simple sugars are progressively converted to complex structural carbohydrates such as cellulose required for plant growth.

Alternatively, the animal can consume an excess of grain or rich hay after escape from a stall or when overfed by an ill-informed caretaker. The food is rich in NSCs, causing bacterial overgrowth in the hind gut and releasing microbial byproducts, generically called "endotoxins," which cause inflammation at distant sites. Any inflammation in the foot is especially damaging in the tight area between the hoof and coffin bone.

Systemic illness, particularly severe infection, also produces powerful systemic activators of inflammation called cytokines. These inflammatory mediators are often causes of secondary, or associated, acute laminitis, as described in some of these case reports.

For some horses, consumption of toxic plants like nightshade, black walnut, and wild cherry leaves and bark will initiate acute laminitis. Other animals appear to be uniquely sensitive to more benign forage like oak leaves.

# Normal Hoof Anatomy and Metabolism

HORSES WALK ON THE ELONGATED middle finger or toe of each leg. They generate a great deal of pressure on each hoof from their body weight and repetitive impacts with the ground. All these forces are transmitted through the continuously growing hoof across to the coffin bone by attachments called laminae. The finger-like projections from the inner surface of the hoof called insensitive laminae interlace with similar projections from the coffin bone (sensitive laminae) and support the forces associated with the horse's gaits (7).

In 1970, during a first-year microscopic anatomy lab in vet school, I saw my first microscope slide of a fetal hoof cross section. That one slide has influenced my approach to every case of laminitis I have treated. The slide of a tiny hoof (about the size of the tip of my little finger) had an impressive network of arteries and veins running up and down every tiny sensitive lamina before the foal was born (its mother had likely died of colic while 7 or 8 months pregnant at the university hospital). The interlacing of primary, secondary, and even tertiary sensitive laminae coming off the coffin bone with corresponding primary, secondary, and tertiary insensitive laminae coming in from the hoof are shown in the artist's drawings. They are very much what I remember.

In horses, each leg receives blood from paired digital arteries. Normally blood flows from the fetlock down through the capillary bed of the hoof, nourishing the sensitive laminae and supporting the metabolic processes necessary for attachment and hoof growth.

Under the microscope tiny arteries have much thicker muscular walls than the corresponding tiny veins. The blood cells move through the arteries under higher pressure before passing single file through the tiny, permeable capillaries to then enter the thin walled, lower pressure veins, then return to the heart and lungs.

The digital arteries also connect in parallel to thick-walled blood vessels in the hoof called arterio-venous anastomoses or AVAs (8), which provide an alternative path for blood to return to the heart. These are pressure relief channels when a horse is galloping. Dr. Pollitt's galloping video (9) shows at the time of maximum weight bearing in the stride, no blood at all may enter the hoof and instead flows though AVAs. The blood pressure spike is relieved which prevents rupture of the fragile capillaries.

Under normal conditions blood flows freely through the capillary bed of the hoof. When more blood is needed in other areas of the body, the large muscular arteries constrict or relax to divert blood to where it is needed.

This very important physiological process is controlled by the sympathetic nervous system. It is why you should not swim soon after eating. Blood has been diverted to your intestines to digest and absorb your meal, but if you swim vigorously, you will need that blood for your arms, so you are much more likely to get a stomachache or muscle cramps.

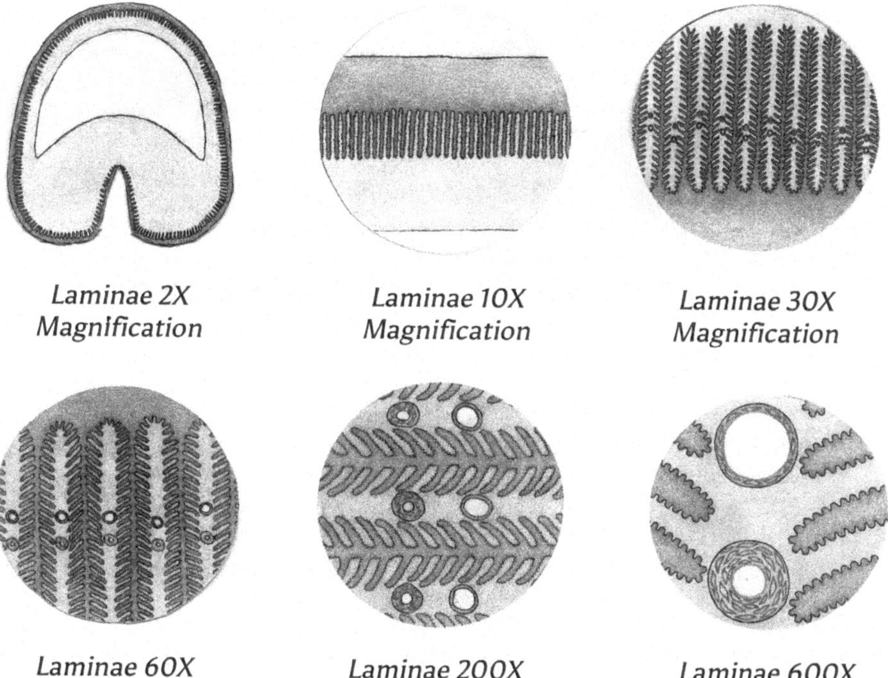

*Laminae 2X Magnification*

*Laminae 10X Magnification*

*Laminae 30X Magnification*

*Laminae 60X Magnification*

*Laminae 200X Magnification*

*Laminae 600X Magnification*

# Inflammation as a Mechanism

## *Edema Impairs Hoof Blood Flow*

ACUTE LAMINITIS BEGINS WHEN INFLAMMATION causes fluid to leak from the capillaries and compress the venous outflow from the hoof. The laminae become ischemic and very painful. The five cardinal signs of inflammation from Greek medicine are heat, pain, swelling, redness, and loss of function. Increased circulation is also common in inflammation, as an attempt to heal a cause of inflammation like damaged or infected cells. In the 1970s and '80s, most vets assumed reduced hoof circulation was inconsistent with inflammation. They dismissed inflammation as a cause of acute laminitis, but increased circulation is not always possible with inflammation within a confined space.

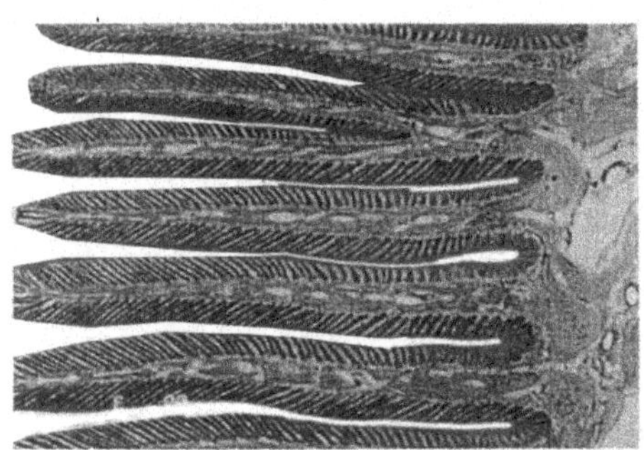

*Acute Laminitis*

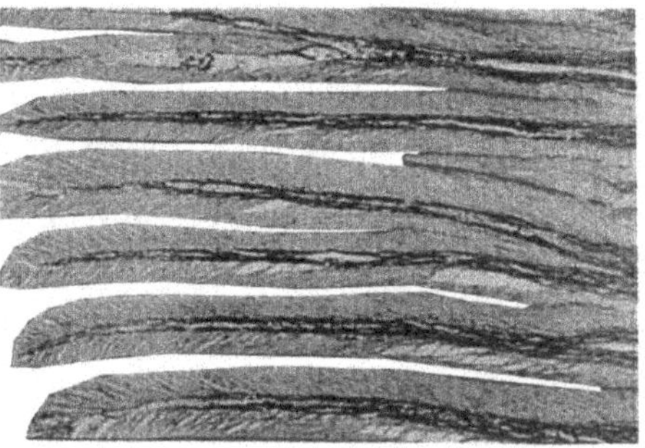

*Normal Laminitis*

The extrinsic pressure from this edema, described by Garner and Coffman, (10) and Hood, (11) squeezes shut the thin laminar veins. The superb photomicrographs from Dr. Chris Pollitt (7) show massive swelling and edema of the insensitive secondary laminae, obliterating the blood flow through the sensitive secondary laminae. Although he has specifically rejected that inflammation is present in acute laminitis, his photographic evidence confirms the presence of the swelling and edema of the insensitive secondary laminae in the first hours of acute laminitis.

Pain and ischemia of the laminae cause reflex vasoconstriction of the smaller arteries in the skin of the shin, fetlock and pastern areas (Figures 3 and 4, left hoof). This raises the systolic digital pulse pressure and increases blood flow downwards, to the hoof. Unfortunately, this increased flow cannot adequately penetrate the tight space between the coffin bone and hoof unless first, there is a reduction of the inflammation and edema.

Researchers for years have incorrectly assumed that these blood vessels have vasoconstricted (11-15). Allen has demonstrated that the relative vascular resistance within the hoof actually shifts during acute laminitis from 92% arterial and 8% venous to 53% arterial and 47% venous (16). Since the veins lack the muscular capability to constrict that the arteries have, vasoconstriction is not the cause of the increased venous resistance. Coffman's angiography (12), Hood's scintigraphy (15) and Pollitt's corrosion casts, (7) all show the same areas of reduced blood flow in laminitis, at the tightest and least flexible hoof and coffin bone attachments.

As blood backs up, the larger arterio-venous anastomoses or AVAs open, bypassing the hoof and producing a bounding digital pulse, palpable just behind the fetlock. Arterial blood flow increases but bypasses the compressed and ischemic capillaries. Although vasoconstriction, AVA shunting and even local blood clots have been postulated as primary inciting factors in acute laminitis (16), they are actually secondary responses to the inflammation and local edema.

Meanwhile, the laminae, under a dual attack of pressure and ischemia, become progressively more painful, making the horse reluctant to move. The immobility further retards blood flow to the hooves. The cycle of pressure which leads to ischemia and pain must be broken early by treating the swelling and edema of inflammation. The increased pulse pressure will decrease or disappear when laminitis is treated and capillary blood flow in the hoof returns to normal.

# Defining Acute Laminitis

**FIRST, I MUST BE CLEAR** that acute doesn't mean severe. Acute defines the first stage of laminitis. This is when the horse first shows pain or bilateral lameness. The horse may exhibit being rocked back on its haunches and refuse to move, or the lameness may be so slight that the inexperienced horseman may not even notice a problem.

## Acute Laminitis Always Precedes Chronic Laminitis

Researchers have repeatedly written that by the time a horse with experimentally induced laminitis first shows pain, there is already permanent damage to his laminae. In more than 40 years treating over 1,200 cases of laminitis in the same suburban Chicago primary care field practice, I have almost never been called to look at a horse with acute laminitis before they show pain. However, I believe every horse with acute laminitis has a window of opportunity for a full cure.

Certainly, the most severe acute cases have a very short window for successful treatment, but the much more common mild acute cases have a much longer window of opportunity for full cure with absolutely no permanent damage, providing they receive treatment as soon as possible.

Acute laminitis, if it is not diagnosed and treated properly, can quickly turn into chronic laminitis (founder) that is almost impossible to fully cure and often leads to a life of pain and misery, with euthanasia all too often the only solution. Many nationally respected equine veterinarians disagree with me. Some have written that they frequently see horses develop chronic laminitis without ever going through the acute stage. They claim these horses have had the very best of care and simply wake up one morning with rotated coffin bones, and absolutely nobody did anything wrong or missed any warning sign of the disease.

Rick Redden, DVM has made a career treating severe founder "train wrecks." I have heard him say at lectures around the country (5,6) that he "has to bury" 90% of the desperate terminal cases sent to his clinic near Lexington, Kentucky. For years he has consulted on and treated extremely expensive horses around the world, apparently saving about 10% of the very worst cases. Dr. Redden wrote in the Annual Proceedings of the American Association of Equine Practitioners (17) that "80% of all acute laminitis cases will be cured with or without treatment, and 20% will fail regardless of treatment chosen." I could not disagree more. Certainly, many horses can recover from mild acute laminitis without treatment (and often without anyone noticing that they had laminitis), but many treatments have been proposed and used the past 40 years that I believe do far more harm than good. To prevent founder and a life of pain or euthanasia, it is essential to recognize, diagnose, and logically treat laminitis in the early stage.

# Encounters with Laminitis

OF THE NEARLY 1,200 CASES of laminitis I have seen, including cases that I had no opportunity to treat in the acute stage, my list of complicated chronic cases now totals 39. Only five of those cases became complicated after I treated them in the acute stage.

Two of the five were ponies hypersensitive to Bute (Butazolidin or phenylbutazone) and died of ulcers within the first 3 to 10 days of treatment. They are discussed in the Bute toxicity report on page 28 of this book.

The third horse had the mildest case of laminitis I've diagnosed. After giving the horse three injections of Bute over 10 days, it was still a touch short-strided, so I referred the horse to a clinic for a second opinion.

My diagnosis was overruled, and the horse was de-nerved for a diagnosis of navicular syndrome. He was sound for about 30 days until the coffin bone came through the sole without further warning.

It remains the worst result I ever saw and the only horse with laminitis that I have ever referred to a hospital or clinic. By comparison, I have referred more than 200 other horses and ponies with lameness issues, colics and assorted illnesses.

My fourth failure was a Standard Bred Stallion (Jet) who died of sub-clinical laminitis although I never examined the horse. My fifth failure was a Quarter Horse that suffered five bouts of laminitis from four different causes in 1990, before the coffin bone dropped without rotating.

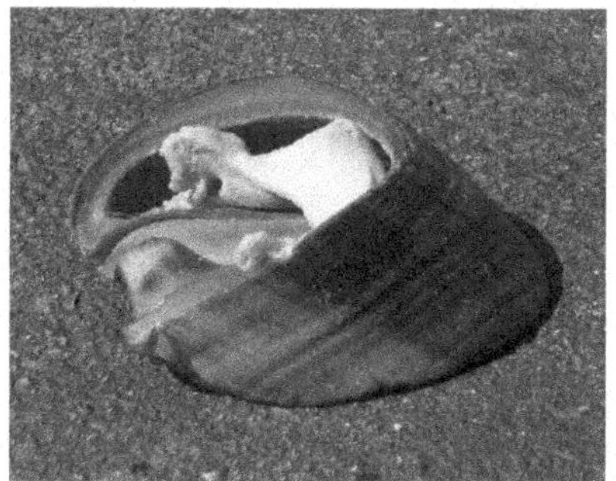

*The coffin bone fits into the hoof cavity.*

*Damaged laminae may cause the snug fit to separate, resulting in a full detachment of the coffin bone and its penetration of the hoof sole.*

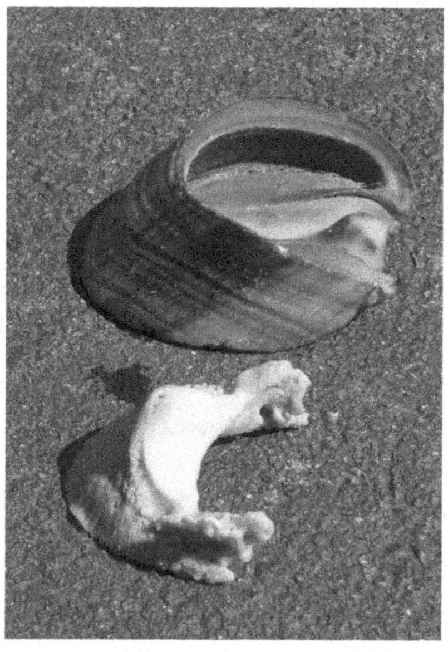

# Beware of SubClinical Laminitis

*It Can Kill Your Favorite Horse*

I HEARD TWO PROFESSORS USE a new term, subclinical laminitis in 2015. Many of my 1,200 actual cases of laminitis fit this new subclinical classification—too slight to diagnose with current technology, invisible to digital X-rays, ultrasound, and even venograms may not show the early signs (18). But it is still capable of causing permanent coffin bone damage, before developing into "clinical" laminitis, and too often leading to permanent lameness or death due to the delayed diagnosis!

At first, I was pleased that they were finally recognizing what I have been warning my clients about. I contacted both these professors, and after verifying their usage of the new term, I was very disappointed that neither had any interest in how I had learned (out of necessity) to diagnose subclinical laminitis. They seem to believe that it cannot be diagnosed with current field technology, but that we now need hospital referrals for MRIs to make the early diagnosis.

I had always considered these mild cases to be primarily undiagnosed, or even worse, misdiagnosed. They were indeed the most dangerous in my private practice.

# Diagnosing Laminitis

EARLY OR EVEN SUBCLINICAL LAMINITIS must be diagnosed with a careful physical exam. First you need to sit back and watch the horse at ease in the stall or cross ties. Does he shift his weight more than normal? Does a normally patient and well-behaved horse ask to pull his foot away from you after 20 seconds of holding it up for cleaning and examination? Or even more telling, does he lift the opposite foot immediately after releasing the foot you were cleaning?

Can you feel an elevated digital pulse pressure after the horse has been standing in his stall or the cross ties for 20 minutes, but then that pulse softens with 3 minutes of walking or trotting in the arena? He might only show occasional slight lameness when turned in figure eights while walking in the barn aisle. The horse may stand normally and trot evenly, but a good rider might tell you he is not reaching out as boldly as he should, "just a little short." Often the owner believes he is "stiff in the shoulders."

I find that hoof testers are unreliable for mild acute laminitis. They are only one test that needs to be considered in early mild cases. The horse may ignore squeezing with the hoof testers, but flinch when tapped on the front of the hoof wall. He might trot off lame on his left front leg after holding up the right front leg for 45 seconds, then switch to lame in the right front side when the left front leg is held up for 45 seconds. He might not have the classic bounding digital pulse, but you might be able to feel a soft pulse behind the front fetlocks that you cannot find behind the hind fetlocks.

If kept in a stall the lameness might only be visible the first couple steps out of the stall, especially when he pivots over a front foot to turn and torques the laminae on the inside foot. You might be able to feel the digital pulse after he has been standing in his stall for an hour, but then not be able to feel it after he has walked just a few minutes. A normally very well-behaved horse might pick his feet up easily for cleaning with a hoof pick or trimming, but slowly start trying to pull it away from you after 45 seconds. It is the foot he is standing on that is starting to hurt after 45 seconds with reduced blood flow to the laminae. Only an observant and educated owner or farrier will make this connection and think sub-clinical mild acute laminitis. This cannot be diagnosed with digital X-rays or ultrasound.

You have to know how to confirm your suspicions by repeating these observations. This requires some degree of sensitivity to your horse if you want to reverse laminitis before your horse founders. There is as much art as science in successful acute laminitis treatment. Constant monitoring of the strength of the digital pulse is my key to determining the intensity and duration of treatment.

# Treating Acute Laminitis

THE PAST QUARTER CENTURY HAS seen more different, and often contradictory, treatments for acute laminitis than for nearly any other equine disease. In every case a triggering cause must be sought, identified and eliminated whether it is spring pasture, alfalfa, excessive grain, obesity, infection or plant toxins such as nightshade, or the medical treatment will fail. Consumption of excess grain or rich pasture can lead to sudden overgrowth of bacteria in the distal colon.

How this triggers laminitis is uncertain, but it may be the most common cause of clinical acute laminitis. I normally give a 1,000-pound horse a gallon of mineral oil via a stomach pump in cases of grain overload or impaction to prevent the development of laminitis.

# Historical Treatments

THE EARLY 20TH CENTURY VETERINARIANS routinely treated acute laminitis by bleeding from the jugular vein, removing the shoes and standing the horse in mud puddles. (3) As late as 1942, the U.S. Department of Agriculture reported that acute laminitis was still "one of the few ailments which may be improved by bleeding…" (19). Bleeding may reduce edema by decreasing the circulating blood volume, but it is certainly not part of modern veterinary practice.

Laminitis research exploded in the early 1970s, but the wide array of currently recommended treatments suggests there is still no consensus regarding treatment. Three of the most recent detailed professional reference texts (20-22) in my personal library include sections on acute laminitis treatment which offer veterinarians menus of 12, 14, and 16 different drugs respectively for treating acute laminitis. I have seen a similarly wide variety of shoeing and trimming suggestions the past 20 years. Remember, "When there are a dozen different treatments for a disease, it is because none of them work really well."

# Conventional Treatment

## *The Vasoconstriction Theory*

IN THE 1970S, A SERIES of radiographic studies (12) showed that the arterioles within the hoof affected by laminitis appeared smaller in diameter than normal. Although laminitis in Latin literally means "inflamed sheets" (laminae), the theory emerged that these narrowed vessels were the result of abnormal constriction of the arterioles. Researchers proposed that laminitis should be treated with powerful vasodilator medications like acepromazine (Ace). The results have been very poor.

Vasodilators such as acepromazine (Ace) cannot act on veins that lack smooth muscle but relax the muscular walls of the arteries, especially the arterio-venous anastomoses (AVAs) at the fetlock. Paradoxically this well-intentioned treatment allows the blood to flow even more rapidly away from the area that needs blood the most.

The opening of the AVAs increases the palpable digital pulses. Vasodilators are still advised in all the equine medical textbooks for the throbbing pulse seen in severe laminitis. This has no benefit when local edema compresses the vessels that deliver blood to the hoof laminae. I have never once used a vasodilator for laminitis, believing it would interfere with the horse's natural mechanism to deliver more blood to his swollen laminae.

# DANGERS OF STALL REST

BECAUSE PAIN IS THE MOST prominent symptom in horses with acute laminitis, current textbooks universally advise complete stall rest for this disease (20-22). The ischemic tissue is so painful the horse is hesitant to walk. But walking is an intrinsic mechanism that normally reduces tissue swelling by pumping out edema fluid trapped between the hoof and coffin bone. Stall rest is actually damaging at this early stage, but too many horses with laminitis are locked in stalls for fear the stressed laminae might tear. You must treat acute laminitis early, when fresh blood can prevent the laminae from becoming weak enough to shear.

Removing the shoes and properly trimming the feet also helps promote the critical circulation. The toes should be short and square to ease break-over and prevent the flexor tendon from pulling the coffin bone away from the weakened laminae. Lowering the heels will aid the pumping action of the hoof.

# A Logical Approach to Treatment

LAMINITIS HAS ALWAYS BEEN THE most predictable disease for me to treat—when I was called early. In every case, the cause of inflammation must be sought and if possible, eliminated. Today, the anti-inflammatory phenylbutazone (Bute) and diuretic furosemide (Lasix or Salix) reduce inflammation and hypertension much more neatly and safely than bleeding. Bute should be repeated daily, decreasing the dosage as the disease recedes but continuing as long as the strength of the digital pulse pressure indicates there is still inflammation within the hoof. Cold water and mud, while messy, are still extremely beneficial for acute Obel Grade III and IV cases, by reducing inflammation and swelling under the hoof. Dr. Pollitt's video (9) shows that removing the shoes and proper trimming greatly improves hoof circulation.

I have never used vasodilators for acute laminitis, but I have always observed a digital pulse pressure drop in response to Bute, cool water and walking without shoes in sand, mud, soft grass or occasionally even snow. I avoid ice because it is so cold it independently causes vasoconstriction and possibly even frostbite injury. There are three serious contraindications for cold hosing and mud treatment. Neither should be used if the coffin bone has already rotated, if the sole is dangerously thin, or if the horse develops pressure abscesses between the sole and coffin bone. In those cases, I prefer to soak with Epsom salts to draw out the edema and wrap the horse's feet in disposable diapers and duct tape. In my practice, unrecognized mild cases are by far the most likely to rotate. All Grade I cases must be taken seriously.

Degree pads are placed between the hoof and shoe by some farriers to elevate the heel and presumably reduce pressure on the coffin bone in an attempt to prevent phalanx rotation. My lone experience with degree pads was when a farrier applied them to a horse with a mild case of laminitis without seeking medical treatment. The horse appeared to be comfortable but rotated 10 degrees before anyone noticed the animal was in trouble.

I prefer to reduce tension on the coffin bone/deep flexor tendon by squaring the toe. Since my intention is to walk the afflicted horse, I almost always lower the heels to promote intermittent frog pressure. This provides a pumping action through the digital cushion (sole) to reduce edema as the horse walks in soft footing. For horses with heels already under run or horses to be stall-rested, I do not necessarily lower the heels.

# The Need for Early Treatment

THIS INTRODUCTION IMPLIES THAT TREATMENT can be so simple that people doubt it can save the difficult cases. I have found severe Obel Grade III and IV cases the easiest to treat because the owners call the quickest and listen the best when their horses are in severe pain. However, I have found mild Grade I or II cases are the most dangerous because owners are apt to delay asking for help. They may take any advice less seriously and the cases are frequently misdiagnosed during the critical first few days.

# Anti-Inflammatory Therapy

### *"Bute"—Phenylbutazone*
### *The Ultimate Double-Edged Sword of Drug Therapy*

BUTE IS A VERY POTENT anti-inflammatory drug with deadly side effects when given in excess. It has a rather narrow therapeutic index, or effective dose versus toxic dose if given for 7 to 10 days (23-26). Multiple texts (20-22) have advised not to give Bute more than 3 consecutive days for acute laminitis. However, the safe use of appropriate doses given for specific medical indications has also been reported for very extended time periods (daily for 6 months with no side effects noted in hundreds of horses) (26).

Using the minimum effective dose of Bute is extremely important to successful treatment of acute laminitis. The safe and effective dosage will change from day to day, horse to horse, and case to case. The horse's owner or trainer who is in charge of monitoring the horse's daily treatment and progress through acute laminitis must be able to assess the changes in comfort and inflammation on a day-to-day basis and adjust the Bute dosage as needed in consultation with the horse's veterinarian.

Used correctly Bute has saved the lives of hundreds of my patients who would have been crippled or killed due to founder. Given in excess it appears to have killed six ponies and two horses in my 42 years of treating thousands of horses with well over 100,000 grams of Bute bought, administered, or prescribed by me personally. The cause of death is usually toxic shock from a perforated ulcer. It is very important to discuss and try to understand each of the two horse and six pony deaths due to the potential side effects of Bute. Bute is the most effective drug for acute laminitis, and given correctly, it is also very safe. Insufficient Bute dosages, whether due to safety concerns or misdiagnosis is one of the leading causes of founder in nearly all chronic laminitis cases I have seen in 42 years.

Asking how much Bute, cold water or walking is sufficient for the typical acute laminitis case is like asking a fireman how much water he uses on a typical fire. Every case of acute laminitis is as different as every fire. You must use as much Bute, water and soft walking as is necessary to keep the digital pulse barely detectable. Any detectable increased digital pulse pressure is an indication of inflammation and cause for continued treatment.

For a 1,000-pound horse, I usually start with 2 grams of Bute IV and then use 2 grams of Bute paste each morning and evening starting on the first day if there is a throbbing pulse. As long as there is any soreness or tendency for the pulse to rebound as the Bute wears off, I am likely to continue using 2 grams of Bute paste twice a day.

When there is substantial improvement, I will drop to 1.5 grams twice a day, then 1 gram once a day as long as the pulse pressure does not return to unacceptable levels. If it does, I raise the Bute dosage back up.

Thin or fit horses with mild and moderate laminitis are generally fully recovered within three to ten days. Severe cases in obese horses usually require six to eight weeks of Bute with decreasing doses as improvement is shown.

All patients must be off Bute at least four days without a significant digital pulse before they may be ridden, worked or shod with discretion.

# Phenylbutazone Overdose or Hypersensitivity

*Bute Toxicity*

DESPITE THE SUSTAINED HIGH DOSES of Bute used to save Sandy McDaniel described in this book, Bute overdose toxicity is a very real possibility (23-25). How much Bute is unsafe? To answer that we must look at each of these horses and ponies who died from Bute. In the Table I have recorded the 4 Shetland ponies, 2 Minis, 2 Welsh ponies, 1 Morgan, and 1 Quarter Horse that died of colic or peritonitis most likely due to Bute caused ulcers. It should be noted that each of the 4 Shetland ponies and the Quarter Horse were all in their 30s. I learned from each of them.

TABLE 1: Bute Toxicity Fatalities (1974 ~ 2016)

| | | | | |
|---|---|---|---|---|
| 1981 | Tigger | 600# | 4 yr Welsh gelding | 24 gm in 12 days |
| 1990 | Charlie | 700# | 24 yr Welsh x Cob gelding | 4 gm in 2 days ~<br>yrs of occasional use |
| 1993 | Tinkerbelle | 500# | 32 yr Shetland mare | 32 gm in 16 days |
| 1998 | Mary | 400# | 33 yr Shetland mare | 1-3 gm daily for about 20 years |
| 2001 | Patches | 400# | 34 yr Shetland gelding | 45 gm in 30 days |
| 2002 | Susie | 1,050# | 10 yr Morgan mare | 28 gm in 6 days |
| 2002 | Rebel | 450# | 36 yr Shetland gelding | 2 gm in 2 days ~<br>yrs of occasional use |
| 2003 | Krystal | 300# | 19 yr Miniature mare | 8 gm in 7 days |
| 2014-15 | Elvis | 400# | 20 yr Shetland gelding | 100 gm in 60-90 days ~<br>10 yrs of occasional use |
| 2006 | Brio | 1,000# | 32 yr AQHA gelding | 20 gm in 45 days |
| 2010 | Ruffo | 400# | Mini | 5 gm in 5 days |

Of the eight Bute fatalities:

- 3 were my fault—over-prescribed for weight of ponies and not sufficiently warned or monitored
- 2 were given Bute by owners without my knowledge
- 2 owners disregarded my instructions and thought if a little helped, more was better
- 1 owner misunderstood my written directions—"1 gm every day or 2" to mean "1 gm or 2 gm each day"
- 3 would have been euthanized 10–20 years earlier without Bute

I had been using as much Bute as necessary to treat laminitis for about ten years before I saw my first Bute induced fatal colon ulcer in a 600-pound Welsh pony. He was only on two grams of Bute a day for eight days when he developed a very profuse diarrhea. He went to the hospital where they euthanized him and told me he had colon ulcers. In retrospect, the 2 grams per day were like giving a 1,200-pound horse 4 grams per day for 8 days, which I would not do unless absolutely needed to save a life. That one was definitely my mistake for the over-dosage.

One of the little Shetlands was on daily Bute for about 20 years with chronic laminitis. She was a great little child's fox hunter and mini eventer with just occasional mild laminitis in the 1970s. Her first few bouts of laminitis were quickly cured with short courses of Bute and pasture reductions. Then she moved out of state for three years with her owner, received different laminitis treatment and came back to Illinois badly foundered. Without Bute she would have been euthanized at least 15 years earlier. Her owners frequently gave up to 3 grams a day despite my repeated warnings that was a dangerously high dosage for such a small pony. Interestingly, long before her repeated colics showed up in her 30s, this pony developed severe arthritis in her knees with very large bone spurs. It became very painful to bend her knees enough to trim her feet her last couple years. I believe the years of Bute interfered with the natural repair and replacement of joint cartilage. However, Bute did give her an extra 15 years with an owner who did not believe in euthanasia for moderate pain.

One other Shetland and the other Welsh pony each died after a single dose of Bute. The two minis died after very short courses of Bute. One of the mini owners misunderstood my written and spoken directions to "give 1 gram Bute every day or two" depending on need (not for laminitis, but for muscle soreness after difficult trimming from an impatient farrier). She gave 2 grams per day and the 300-pound mini was toxic within the week. Neither of the two horses who died from Bute ever had laminitis. The Morgan died after just a week of overdoses by her owner due to a misdiagnosis and excessive Bute before she was even seen by a vet. The Quarter Horse was 33, and he only received about 15 grams of Bute over 30 days (never more than 1 gram in a day) for a severe eye ulcer. His perforated colon ulcer was likely caused as much by the stress of losing his sight in the eye and getting unfairly bullied by a new horse in his pasture.

While ponies made up only about 10% of my patients, and maybe 20% of my laminitis cases, they accounted for 80% of my Bute toxicity. It must be noted that perfectly normal ponies were used in the research trials in testing for Bute toxicity. I consider 1 gram of Bute to be an overdose for a pony with no active inflammation. My practical experience indicates that Bute works at the site of active inflammation, before excess Bute might attack the intestinal lining causing ulcers. The key is to customize the treatment to give enough, but not too much, and that can change daily according to the pain, inflammation, and other treatments! I always advise the "Minimum-Effective" dose of Bute with adjustments made daily based on the horse's needs and response to treatment.

Extrapolating from my typical yearly purchases of Bute, over 42 years I prescribed well over 100,000 grams of Bute to more than 2,000 horses and ponies. About 1,200 of those prescriptions were for laminitis. For my practice, the benefits of Bute in acute laminitis appear to outweigh the risks 100 to 1, when used at the minimum effective daily dose. The potential ulceration is reversible if monitored, but chronic laminitis (founder) cannot be fully reversed.

My theory of laminitis has always differed from the professors and researchers; and after my first ten years, it was obvious I was getting much different results from what they predicted for laminitis. So, I started tracking my laminitis cases in 1984. The failures are much easier to remember, and much more significant learning experiences. I have included here more than fifty laminitis cases, each of which was different in presentation, but very similar in results. If diagnosed early and treated logically they recover very nicely and quickly return to full use. If diagnosis is delayed or treatment is based on severe symptoms rather than the abnormal physiology, far too many crash. In my practice, the severity of the initial pain was inversely related to the end result. My clients would call much quicker, and they listened much better when their horses were in sudden severe pain.

When it became apparent that I would not develop a statistically significant data base by recording only the failures, I started recording every case, and I am now past 1,200. These are simply "anecdotes" to the researchers, but they are evidence to practitioners like me. We have to make practical treatment decisions every day based on the evidence we see in front of us on that day.

Very few veterinarians report or even track their less famous failures, but published papers have reported a fatality rate at close to 50% for several university hospitals (28). Some of these horses come in badly foundered, but too many others develop laminitis while in the hospital for other reasons. Another published report showed that a university field veterinarian who focused on testing all his laminitis patients for Cushing's disease lost 25% of his on-the-farm laminitis patients to founder over his 4-year study (29). An extensive survey of farms across the country reported just 6% of laminitis patients dying (mostly treated by private practitioners) (30). I have only had to euthanize 26 horses (and ponies) due to uncontrolled founder in 42 years. That is just over 2%, but most importantly, every one of my laminitis fatalities was due to human error and delayed diagnosis, never "the mysterious nature of the disease," which is always blamed for the famous fatalities.

Some might say that my 1,200 cases are inflated because many of them were what they now call subclinical. In fact, nearly all the fatalities were missed in the "subclinical" stage. That is when laminitis is the easiest to cure. Laminitis that is subclinical is just as real as subclinical pregnancy, subclinical cancer, or subclinical heart disease in humans. How many days, weeks, or months of a head start do you want to give laminitis before making a correct diagnosis? Treatment must be logical and timely, never symptomatic and delayed.

Acute laminitis is an emergency. Every day the horse goes without optimum circulation to his laminae he is at risk of permanent laminar damage. Founder is the result of unrecognized or unsuccessfully treated acute laminitis. Acute has nothing to do with severity. It is merely the early stage of the disease—severe or mild—before coffin bone movement has started. That is when founder must be prevented with early intervention, not symptomatic treatment. The cause(s) must be identified and eliminated, and the owners must take my advice seriously in the mild cases. They listen very well in the severe cases.

I initially prepared the following two clinical papers ten years ago for academic publication. The papers have not been published and are presented here to support my long-standing convictions about the etiology and treatment of acute laminitis. "The Seasonality of Laminitis," followed by "A 42-Year Clinical Trial, Treating Acute Laminitis as Vasocompression, Never Vasoconstriction (1974-2016)."

Immediately following are my stories of horses with laminitis that illustrate the range of acute laminitis symptoms and the treatment combinations needed to obtain an optimal outcome.

# The Seasonality of Laminitis

*David Frederick, DVM*

THERE WERE TWO PEAKS OF laminitis episodes during the study period, one in May-June and the other in August-September. In these four months, the laminitis incidence was 50% greater than the mean incidence for the other 8 months. This suggests a link between the pasture growth and laminitis risk for this period in Northern Illinois.

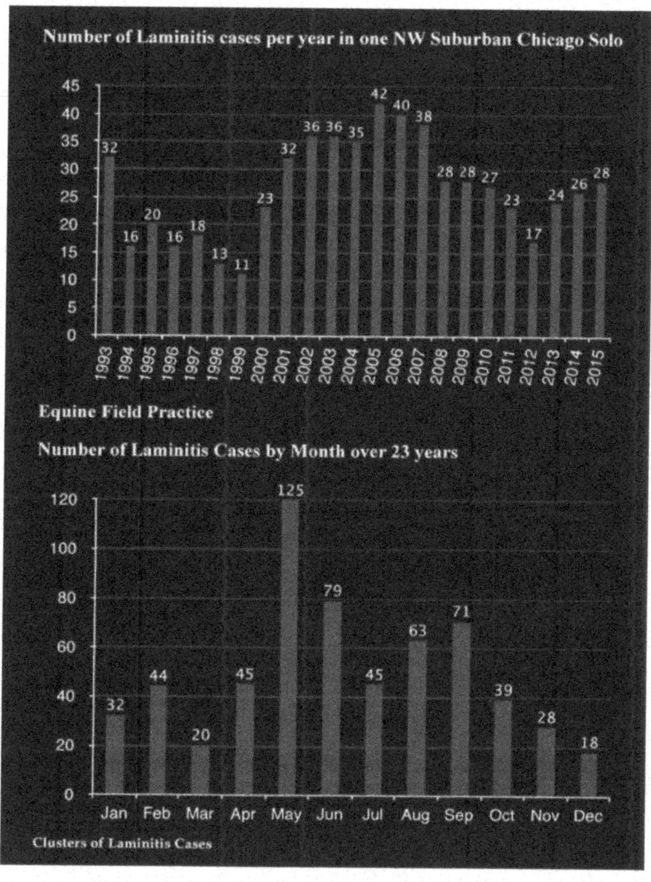

# A 42-Year Clinical Trial of Vasocompression, Not Vasoconstriction

## *120 Worst of 1,200+ Cases Investigated (1974-2016)*

David Frederick, DVM

Having seen severe acute laminitis treated simply, quickly, and dramatically in 1968, prior to entering veterinary school, I have held a minority theory on the pathogenesis and effective treatment of acute laminitis my entire career (1974-2016) in the same solo, suburban, equine field practice, northwest of Chicago, Illinois. I absolutely disagree with Dr. Chris Pollit's statement: "From the outset it must be understood that a therapeutic regime, using biological or chemotherapeutic agents able to arrest or block the triggering of laminitis, does not exist.(1)" The same pre-eminent researcher has also written that "Some fortunate horses experience the foot pain of acute laminitis, but do not develop distal phalanx displacement and appear to make a complete recovery."(1) I have treated about 1,080 milder laminitis patients, not analyzed for this paper, who have made complete recoveries from the clinical pain of acute laminitis.

Starting in 1984, following Burney Chapman's address to the American Association of Equine Practitioners on radical hoof resections and heart bar shoes as a salvage procedure for chronic laminitis or founder (2), I have retrospectively tabulated all my complicated, or severe acute Grade IV laminitis cases from the years 1974 to 1992. In 1984, all serious cases of laminitis seen the first 10 years of practice were reconstructed using medical records, and information recalled by this author and his clients. I treated all severe or complicated cases with a consistent protocol to treat the vasocompression of compartment syndrome caused by inflammation and edema within the hard hoof capsule. A conflicting theory presumes that laminitis is caused by vasoconstriction of blood vessels in the hoof. None of my patients were ever given a vasodilator, which I have always believed would be contraindicated.

From 1993 to 2016, all cases of laminitis were recorded in real time. A significant number of these horses were treated differently by other veterinarians prior to becoming my patients. Others had subsequent relapses after their owners moved out of state and were treated to relieve presumed vasoconstriction causing laminitis. I have made a serious effort to identify and tabulate the causes and mistakes which led to all complicated cases and the most dramatic recoveries. The 120 worst or most severe cases (out of approximately 1,200 total) were analyzed. The other approximately 1,080 cases recovered very quickly and could be considered routine, but it is precisely those types of cases that are too often ignored by the owners during the "window of opportunity." I believe every laminitis case has such a window to reverse the disease and prevent damage, if diagnosed early and treated logically, rather than symptomatically.

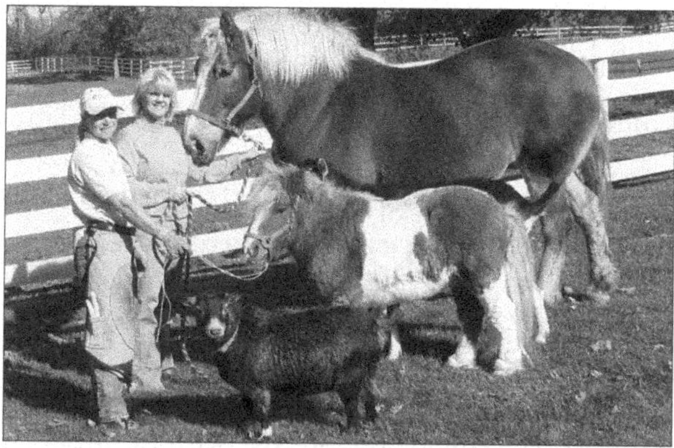

*This Belgian mare represents 5 of the 120 most serious cases selected that were Belgian mares with retained placentas.*

*The Standard pony had a Grade IV flare up of Chronic Laminitis 10 years in a row, always in August and September due to pasture and hyper-sensitivity to falling walnut leaves, yet ran Bute-free the other 10 months.*

Twenty-six of the 1,200 cases were eventually euthanized due to permanent lameness. Seven ponies died of probable phenylbutazone toxicity, either inadvertent overdose or hypersensitivity.

- 2 Miniature Horses
- 3 Shetland ponies
- 2 Welsh
- 0 horses with laminitis died of Bute toxicity
- 1 horse which never had laminitis died of Bute toxicity
- 56 of the 1,200 horses and ponies died or suffered permanent career changing damage
- 14 horses suffered significant damage but were "pasture sound" without drugs
- 2 horses and 1 pony lived on daily Bute the rest of their lives
- 7 horses died of concurrent disease, not due to their laminitis
- 64 of the most serious cases and all 1,080 milder cases returned to previous use with very brief and uneventful treatment
- 19 horses returned to their previous use despite significant hoof damage
- 22 horses returned to their previous use with minimal visible hoof changes
- 23 horses recovered from severe Grade III or IV Acute Laminitis with no visible damage

The most likely causes of the laminitis in the 120 horses and ponies analyzed in this study were identified in every case—usually between 2 and 5 causes for every case. It is extremely important to identify and correct all causes.

74 Alfalfa Hay — 5 Retained Placenta

60 Excessive Grain — 3 Road Concussion

59 Lush Pasture — 2 Dexamethazone

41 Clover — 2 Corn

41 Excessive Stall time — 2 Walnut Leaves and Bark

33 "Easy Keepers" — 2 Abscesses

26 Cushing's (PPID) Signs and Symptoms — 1 Colic

15 Equine Metabolic Syndrome or Obesity — 1 West Nile Virus

13 Nightshade — 1 Vitamin K-3 Kidney Failure

6 Wild Cherry Tree Leaves or Bark — 1 Oak Leaves

Human errors contributed to virtually all the failures analyzed (Table 2 on page 40). 58 times the owner made serious errors. 14 times I made significant mistakes—usually not recognizing very mild laminitis, allowing some of the ponies to be overdosed with Bute, and using acute treatments too far into chronic, unstable cases. 30 times a previous vet made serious errors, and the horses were well into the chronic stage before the author saw them. 11 times a subsequent vet treated vasoconstriction rather than vasocompression with poor results. 6 times a trainer made errors. And just 2 farriers failed to recognize acute laminitis. 2 other farriers used inappropriate treatments.

## TABLE 2
## ANALYSIS OF HUMAN ERRORS
## *(120 episodes)*

| | |
|---|---|
| Owner errors | 58 |
| My errors | 14 |
| Previous vet errors | 30 |
| Subsequent vet errors* | 11 |
| Trainer errors | 6 |
| Farrier errors | 4 |
| Missed laminitis | 2 |
| Inappropriate treatment | 2 |

*Missed diagnosis or treated with inadequate Bute, stall confinement, IV fluids, and vasodilators

# Discussion

**THERE IS NO MORE CONSENSUS** on effective treatment of acute laminitis today than there was 100 years ago, and it is most unfortunate for horses. In 1903, Dr. Dennis Magner wrote, "The first or acute stage can be invariably cured which is not at all difficult to do; the second, or chronic, stage is not curable, but may be palliated to a limited extent." (3) Dr. Caulton Reeks, a British professor, and Fellow of the Royal College of Veterinary Surgeons, had frustratingly different opinions on laminitis treatment in his classic 1906 book, *Diseases of the Horse's Foot.* (4) In the *1907 USDA Report on Diseases of the Horse* there was simply one sentence on treatment of laminitis: "The treatment of laminitis is probably more varied than in any other disease, and yet a large number of cases recover for even the poorest practitioner." (5) The 1942 revision of the USDA report warned, "Bleeding, both general and local, should be guarded against." (6) But the 1942 *Yearbook of Agriculture* also published by the USDA, stated that acute laminitis was still, "one of the few ailments which may be improved by bleeding…" (7)

In 1986 and 1988, Dr. Ric Redden stated at the AAEP Conventions that 20% of all laminitis cases become complicated "regardless of therapy" and 80% remain non-complicated, "with or without treatment." (8,9) I absolutely do not agree that any percentage of acute laminitis cases are doomed to fail due to, "the mysterious nature of the disease." Practicing medicine is very much like professional sports, in so far as the need to improve our skill by analyzing and correcting our mistakes. We can learn far more from our failures than from our successes. There is far too much peer pressure to not discuss mistakes for fear of litigation. The silence might be good business for veterinarians, but it hurts the horses we need to help.

My basic belief, that the swelling and edema of inflammation within a confined space, is what causes the lack of circulation to the laminae, has never changed. I have believed since veterinary school that the increased digital pulse pressure seen with laminitis is the horse's sympathetic nervous system response to anoxia in the laminae. The horse must have "acute, oxygen-sensing mechanisms" in the laminae similar to the human oxygen-sensing mechanisms described by Weir in the *New England Journal of Medicine* in 2005. (10) This sympathetic nervous system attempt to restore adequate circulation to the laminae should not be interfered with by veterinarians with vasodilators, stall confinement, and therapeutic shoes in the acute stage of laminitis. Time is critical depending on the severity of the inflammation. Horses with mild inflammation, allowed to roam, and with good hoof conformation may heal themselves if the cause is removed, but severe inflammation has a very short window of opportunity for correct treatment.

I have seen this simple treatment work in some very sick horses while they were dying of peritonitis, kidney failure, and West Nile disease. The reason there is a much higher fatality rate for laminitis in hospitals is mainly due to stall confinement in the acute stage and the tendency to use more vasodilators, and IV fluids, but less phenylbutazone and Lasix.

Laminitis must be treated as an emergency more like human strokes and heart attacks. Restoring the circulation as soon as possible can make all the difference between success and failure. Locking a horse with acute laminitis in a stall and waiting to see what will happen due to the "mysterious nature of the disease" is unacceptable.

Horses cannot wait for unethical and inhumane "double blind trials" for laminitis. We need to recognize what works and try to understand why it works. There has already been an abundance of incredibly good research published, but it has been interpreted incorrectly. I used Dr. Pollitt's photomicrographs and corrosion casts 15 years ago to explain laminar edema causing vasocompression within the hoof and the horse compensating with vasoconstriction outside the hoof. Sadly, he still does not agree, and too many horses continue to die. (11)

# References (For Pages 36-42)


1. Pollitt C., *Equine Laminitis*. RIRDC, 2001.
2. Chapman B, Platt G., Proceedings Am Assoc Equine Pract. 1984; 30:99.
3. Magner D., *Magner's Standard Horse and Stock Book*. 1905:409 and 492.
4. Reeks HC., *Diseases of the Horse's Foot*. 1906.
5. Holcombe AA., "Special Report on Diseases of the Horse," USDA. 1907:414-430.
6. Holcombe AA., "Special Report on Diseases of the Horse," USDA. revised 1942 by Giltner LT. 426.
7. Mott LO, et al., *Yearbook of Agriculture*. USDA, 1942; 456.
8. Redden R., Proceedings Am Assoc Equine Pract. 1986; 32:648.
9. Redden R., Proceedings Am Assoc Equine Pract. 1988; 34:312.
10. Weir EK., "Acute Oxygen-Sensing Mechanisms." *N Engl J Med*, Nov. 10, 2005; 353:19; and Mar. 2, 2006; 354:9.
11. Frederick D., *American Farriers Journal*. Sept/Oct 1997.

# ~SECTION I~

## A Very Mild Case, Recognized and Treated Properly

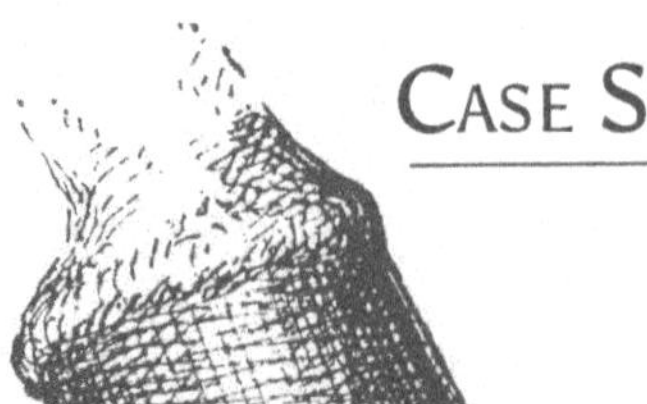

# Case Study

## "Surprise"

### *Laminitis Myths and Mistakes*

WHEN FAMOUS HORSES LIKE BARBARO, Secretariat, Affirmed, Nihilator, and Dash for Cash have been euthanized due to laminitis, the disease is usually described as a "mysterious," "incurable," and "often fatal," disease by both the mainstream media and horse publications. Even peer reviewed professional veterinary journals have published scientific articles frankly stating there is "no cure for laminitis," and laminitis researchers like to claim, "by the time the horse shows pain from laminitis, there has already been permanent damage" done to his feet. Each of the five famous horses listed above had access to some of the most prestigious, intelligent, educated, and seriously experienced equine veterinarians in the world. If a horse is "lucky" enough to survive laminitis, university clinicians will warn everyone that a laminitis survivor will live with the consequences of the disease the rest of his life, requiring "lifelong special shoeing," expensive "special management," and often daily medication for a reasonably comfortable, "pasture sound" life.

The popular press never, and trade publications rarely distinguish between acute and chronic laminitis. Occasionally peer reviewed scientific journals also ignore the distinction when discussing the prognosis and treatment of laminitis. This distinction is critical to understanding the disease, which the laminitis research industry claims is a great mystery, despite having been the subject of hundreds of published research articles the past 35 years and dozens of laminitis specific professional conferences the past 20 years.

By definition, the medical term "acute," refers to the first stages of a disease, which may be hours, days, or sometimes weeks, before a disease becomes chronic, due to relatively permanent, disease-related, pathologic changes in the tissues affected. In laminitis, the shift from acute to chronic occurs when there is either rotation or sinking of the coffin bone within the hoof. This movement of the coffin bone stretches and tears the oxygen deprived and sensitive laminae. In severe cases the acute phase may be shockingly short (sometimes less than 24 hours from when the severe acute phase starts), whereas in mild cases, it can easily stretch for a week or more, unnoticed, without any permanent damage. Proper diagnosis and treatment in the acute phase is critical for full success in severe cases. Mild cases may heal themselves if the lameness is recognized, the cause removed, and the horse has sufficient room to roam on reasonably trimmed feet.

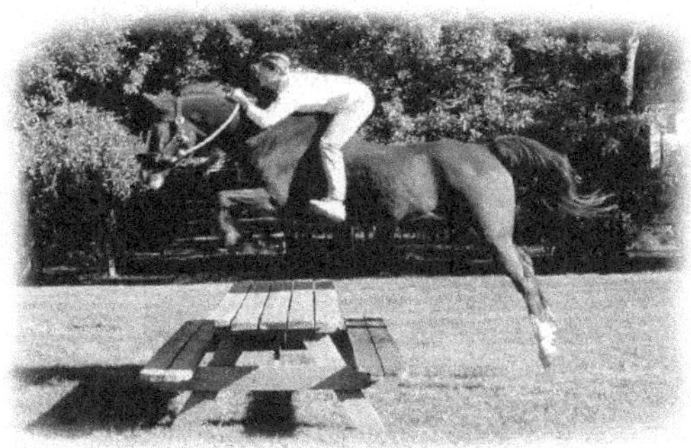

*Surprise and My Wife Julie*
*Entertaining the Family*

Surprise was my wife Julie's, Arab x AQHA jumper gelding, whom I had helped her feed and care for on a daily basis since he was a yearling. Surprise was the perfect eventing, fox hunting, driving, and family horse for 33 years. His medical history repeatedly contradicts some of the more blatant myths perpetrated about laminitis. I have helped cure him of acute laminitis at least seven times since the early 1980s, yet the spring of 2007 was the only time I ever saw even the slightest separation of his white line. In addition to his seven or more episodes of acute laminitis, Surprise probably spent the night with our grain barrel tipped over a couple dozen times in the 33 years we had him.

Laminitis is even easier to prevent than to cure. Only once did Surprise develop even mild acute laminitis after eating 20 to 40 pounds of grain in the middle of the night. Nearly always his access to a night of free choice grain was from jumping out of pastures, fiddling with gates, or opening large sliding, but unlocked, double barn doors. He was only rarely kept in a stall the night before an early morning fox hunt, combined training event, pony club rally for our daughter, or on severe weather nights (10 below zero is not as severe as 30 degrees above zero with freezing rain).

When Surprise had eaten 20 to 40 pounds of grain he tipped over, my standard next morning treatment was usually 12cc of dipyrone (a medication to relax his intestine), 2gm of Bute IV to prevent inflammation, a gallon of mineral oil to speed the passage and reduce the absorption of the endotoxins caused by grain overload, no grain, alfalfa, clover, or lush pasture for a couple days, and at least 48 hours turnout to maintain the circulation in his hooves. When given this early prophylactic treatment, he never developed even mild laminitis from his periodic grain binges. In fact, in 40 years of private primary care equine field practice and approximately 1,200 cases of laminitis from all causes, I have never had any horse develop laminitis after a night of gorging in an open grain barrel whenever the owners have called the next morning for my standard laminitis prevention protocol. Those who failed to call in the morning, when they found their loose horse in the grain overnight, have, sometimes, had their horses develop laminitis within 48 hours. As long as these owners called at the first sign of lameness, their horses also invariably responded promptly to effective logical treatment and were cured of the acute laminitis.

I should mention here that my wife has never been shy about expressing, and staunchly defending, her opinions when they have differed from mine. Very fortunately she learned my minority view about the early treatment of laminitis as a young Pony Clubber before we ever met. She first heard about laminitis from an instructor who had spent her summers in the 1950s on her grandmother's horse farm near the University of Pennsylvania's New Bolton Center. Although nearly all vet schools now currently teach mandatory stall confinement, her first memories of laminitis as a child were, "you have to get them walking, even though it hurts!"

Now, I mentioned Prize did develop acute laminitis just once after a night with free choice grain. That happened in September 1990 while my wife and I were on a week's pilgrimage to Medjugore, Yugoslavia. We had left Prize with a client whose own horse had ironically had two separate bouts of laminitis that spring. Prize, a very easy keeper at that time, was being left in the paddock outside the barn at night with the client's horse, who was also an easy keeper.

Their large sliding barn door was shut, but not locked. Prize, as he often liked to try just in case someone forgot, slid the door open, found the grain barrel like a mouse finds cheese, tipped it over until the lid popped off and shared his buffet with his new friend. It happened to be Friday night, and when my client found the remains of the mess Saturday morning, the horses acted perfectly fine, so she did not call another vet. She decided, since she would be home over the weekend, she would just watch the horses to wait and see if the grain was going to be a problem.

The horses reportedly seemed fine all day Saturday and Sunday, but by Monday morning (48 hours since finding the horses had eaten the grain) the client's horse was obviously developing laminitis again. That year the client had been through this twice earlier with that horse, so she knew enough to start her horse back on Bute before leaving for work Monday morning. Since we were due back on Tuesday, she still did not call a backup vet.

We heard about the Friday night grain raid when we went to pick up Prize the following Tuesday evening. The client's horse was still obviously sore despite two days of Bute, but "much better" according to the owner who thought he was coming along just fine. Prize walked fine also, but when I reached down to check his digital pulse pressure, it was very easy to find and obviously stronger than normal. Prize's feet responded very promptly to a couple days of Bute, and no damage was done. His last sliding barn door/grain barrel incident was Christmas morning 2007, when my wife forgot to double lock our barn door after a very late Christmas Eve feeding and turnout.

I have written notes regarding Surprise's last four brief bouts with laminitis that started on June 6, 2003, April 19, 2004, June 5, 2004, and October 3, 2006. I remember one or two other very similar bouts when he was competing in the

1980s that I didn't bother to document at the time (since I've never sent bills to my wife). In the 1980s, Prize worked seriously and steadily, lived in very good pastures, and was fed whatever grain he needed to keep him in good flesh for eventing. The amount changed frequently according to his work, the weather, the pasture growth, and the quality of the hay at the time. Prize was always an exceptionally sound horse, but at least twice in those years he developed bilateral front foot soreness with readily detectable digital pulses. Both times we backed off the grain and good pasture, gave him Bute for a couple days, and he was perfect and back to work within the week.

The last four bouts with laminitis came at a different stage in Prize's life. He showed progressive signs of Cushing's syndrome (caused by an excess production of corticosteroids) for 15 to 20 years by shedding more slowly every year. He became much harder to keep weight on in his mid-20s. Despite regular, conservative, non-power floating dentistry, his molars started wearing out in his early 20s to the point where he had to work very hard to chew hay his last ten years. He still loved to jump. In fact, he jumped out of his good pasture about eight times the summer of 2006 (at age 30!). One day after a short dressage workout that summer, to back up my bragging to a friend about what Prize could still do after most horses have died of "old age," Julie jumped him over a full-sized picnic table. Jumping the picnic table became an annual event with cameras ready (repeated at ages 31, 32, 33, and 34!). Anyway, we had to give Prize two large coffee cans (about 7 or 8 pounds) of Senior pellets mixed with sweet feed (and cracked corn in the winter when there was no edible pasture) twice a day to keep his ribs and hips covered with reasonable flesh.

On the first three dates listed above, 7 to 8 pounds of rich grain, twice a day, while on good pasture, proved to be too much as my wife would inform me that he was "off," and I'd find the increased digital pulse pressure in his front feet, but not the rear. Sometimes we could verify his laminitis by watching his discomfort increase when turned around after walking down the barn aisle. Turning in the aisle torques the sensitive laminae and may be the only sign of laminitis when walking. In the milder cases we could also verify pain in both front feet by merely holding up a front foot and watching him trot off slightly lame in the foot he was asked to stand on for 45 seconds. The hoof testers might show very slight differences in sensitivity through his excellent hoof wall and sole, but I could easily elicit a flinch by tapping sharply on his front hoof walls which that he would ignore on the rear hooves. Only the last time, October of 2006 (at age 30), was his acute laminitis severe enough that I noticed it first myself when he was leaving his stall after breakfast. Every time we treated him with Bute for a few days, backed off the grain, and he was fine within a week.

Some people say these mild cases can't be compared to the severe cases of famous horses previously mentioned. In my practice, as in Prize's last case, it is the mild cases which the owners frequently don't notice or delay calling the vet, that are much more likely to suffer some rotation before the vet is called. When the horses are in severe, sudden pain the owners call very quickly, and we see that their horses are treated as quickly as a colic emergency.

The point of Prize's six bouts of acute laminitis is that every chronic disease is preceded by the acute disease, and that is when laminitis can be most fully cured. The length of the window of opportunity for full cure is (the "golden hour" for human stroke and heart attack victims) directly related to the severity of the attack. More severe attacks need to be treated with the same urgency as human strokes or heart attacks. Sensitive laminae, fully deprived of oxygen, can fail very quickly. Merely decreased oxygen supply from more moderate laminar swelling (inflammation within the confined space between the hoof and coffin bone) takes longer to damage the laminae, but it still must be recognized and corrected.

These mild cases are very easy to miss in their early stages. In Prize's first five episodes my wife, who rode him almost daily, would inform me that he just "wasn't right." She rode him well over 10,000 times (365 days/year x 33 years + 8 leap days = 12,045 days!) since he was a two-year-old. Julie could feel when he wasn't right, even if the vet/husband couldn't see it. Good riders and drivers can often feel what a vet can't see, and then the vet has to examine the horse more closely. Technology is no help in diagnosing acute laminitis. By the time there is diagnostic rotation on radiographs, the horse is into the chronic stage. Blood tests tell you nothing conclusive about acute laminitis. The vet must diagnose acute laminitis solely with the physical exam. Often the history is only revealed by hard questioning and serious inspection of the feed and pasture. The cause must be found and eliminated.

While severe acute laminitis can be obvious by the horse's strained stance or refusal to pick up either front foot, the horse with mild acute laminitis may show little reluctance to pick up a foot, stand absolutely normally, and show very little reaction to hoof testers. These horses need to be checked very carefully for slight increases in digital pulse pressure in the front feet versus the same horse's rear feet. Like humans, the horse has "oxygen sensors" which feed the sympathetic nervous system to constrict less vital skin vessels and redirect blood flow when there is a local oxygen deficit in the laminae (27).

Most all veterinarians were incorrectly taught in school to symptomatically treat the palpably increased digital pulse pressure felt in acute laminitis with vasodilators such as acepromazine or nitroglycerine. I have always believed that was wrong, and I have never used either for laminitis. Stall confinement and special shoes are also widely recommended, but I believe both are more often harmful than helpful for restoring optimum circulation with acute laminitis. Some think the deep flexor tendon pulls the coffin bone way from the laminae, so they either raise the heels, or sever the flexor tendon. I disagree. The laminae fail due to cellular weakness from a lack of oxygen. The best way to correct that is to reduce the inflammation ASAP. Allow the horse to walk freely and gently on properly trimmed feet (low heels, squared toe), on soft ground (not concrete aisles or gravel driveways, and certainly not in box stalls (where every second step requires a pivoting/twisting turn). And identify and remove the most likely cause(s) of the flare-up.

With prompt and correct treatment, there is no percentage of acute laminitis cases that need to fail, "due to the nature of the disease." The basics of laminitis are no different from the basics of heart attacks and strokes. You must restore the optimum circulation ASAP for full recovery from acute laminitis. When heart attacks and strokes are caught early, treated correctly (within the "Golden Hour"), and fully cured, some people like to think the patient must not have really had a heart attack or stroke since there was no visible damage done. I wonder if such people would like their cancer not detected until it's really obvious to everyone. Early detection and correct treatment is just as important with laminitis.

I mentioned that Prize's most recent bout of laminitis was the only one I noticed first as he was leaving his stall after breakfast on October 3, 2006. That episode required Bute for five days before my wife said he felt perfectly solid trotting again. Whereas his previous five episodes were each cured with just two or three doses of Bute. He looked fine all winter following that incident. However, when I got around to trimming his feet on March 17, 2007, for the first time ever he had some separation in his white line. It was five months before I realized that the reason I was the first to notice Prize's latest laminitis was because my wife, an international flight attendant, had been traveling when I noticed Prize was off walking out of his stall. After treating Prize on October 6th, my notes actually indicated that Prize looked to me like he could have been "a little off coming out of his stall" on Tuesday October 3rd, and on Wednesday October 4th he just looked noticeably like a "very old horse" leaving his stall after breakfast. Yet when I watched him in the field those two days he looked fine, and he came into the barn quite solid. It wasn't until Thursday, October 5th after Julie returned home and rode him, that she demanded I check him more carefully. If she had been home earlier in the week, she likely would have felt the laminitis a couple days before I saw it. Nevertheless, with 2 grams of Bute for three days, then 1 gram for two more days, and a temporary grain reduction, he felt absolutely normal within a week.

It wasn't until five months later that I saw the first white line separation, not at his toe, but at the outside wall of his left front and left hind hooves. While the slight separation has had no effect whatsoever on Prize's soundness (he continued to jump the picnic table each of the next four summers at ages 31, 32, 33, and 34!), it was physical evidence that the 72-hour delay from when I first noticed he was off as he left his stall until I examined him and made the diagnosis was sufficient to alter his laminar architecture for the only time in his life.

Why didn't I check him more carefully at the first sign? When Julie was traveling, I typically just opened the barn door twice a day, Prize walked into his stall for grain, and I let him out the same way closing the door behind him as he returned to the pasture. Prize walked absolutely fine coming into the barn those days. It was only leaving his stall after being in eating and waiting maybe an hour for me to return and let him out that he showed anything. By the time I saw the soreness he was walking out the door without a halter. Coming back in the next time he would look fine again, then be off leaving the stall again. The stall time didn't cause the laminitis, but it certainly contributed enough to reducing the circulation and increasing the discomfort that I should have realized what was happening before my wife returned from her trip.

Some veterinarians claim that some horses can rotate and become chronic without going through the acute stage. Their state of denial may make themselves and their clients feel better, but it does nothing for the horses, or for the under- standing of laminitis. Most chronic diseases are preceded by the acute disease. Many diseases are hard to notice in the mild early stages. Cancer and heart disease are great examples. The owner must call the vet when laminitis is in the acute stage, and the vet must diagnose it correctly, treat correctly, and identify and remove the most likely cause(s). The proper treatment must be continued until the horse is fully healed. Stopping Bute after three days because it could cause an ulcer is just as wrong as locking these horses in a stall. Bute must be given at the minimum effective dose until the horse is cured. This is often less than a week in mild cases with lean or fit horses, but it will typically take four to six weeks of decreasing Bute doses in fat horses with more severe symptoms.

Laminitis is no more mysterious than flying an airplane. Only by recognizing and admitting our mistakes can we prevent them the next time. Those who prefer to remain in denial are doomed to repeat their mistakes.

# ~SECTION II~

## Very Mild Early (SubClinical?) Cases that Die

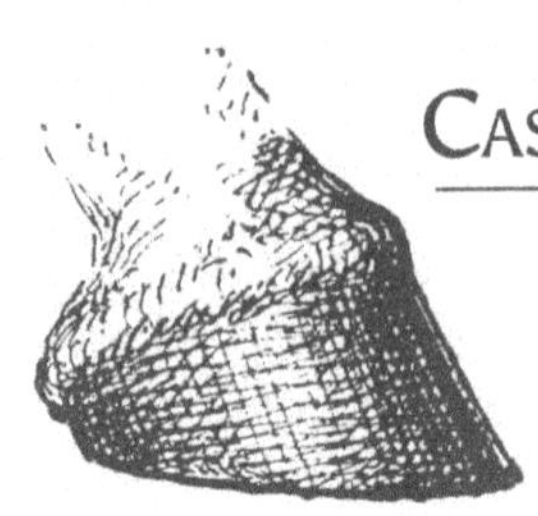

## Case Study

# "Peter" and "Jet"

*Two extremely mild, but misdiagnosed and fatal cases of acute laminitis*

WE ALL LIKE TO HEAR and read dramatic stories with happy endings, but often veterinarians learn the hardest lessons from boring stories with sudden, tragic endings. In 1979 and 1989, I saw two of the mildest cases of acute laminitis ever, and both horses died because of the worst mistakes I have ever made with laminitis. (Over the past 42 years I've made plenty of other serious mistakes with colics, foalings, infections, and lamenesses. The point is to try to learn as we practice medicine.) Ironically, I was joined in these two laminitis cases by nationally prominent, and much more experienced veterinarians who also failed to recognize the early signs of fatal laminitis. Of the 1,200 more obvious cases of acute laminitis or chronic laminitis flare-ups the past 42 years, I've only had to euthanize two others in addition to the two horses described here. Every fatal case I have been involved with was due to human error, not the "mysterious nature of the disease." I wrote up these two cases many years ago, but no journal or magazine has been interested in publishing my "anecdotes."

On June 5, 1979, I was called to look at Peter, a retired 17-year-old Quarter Horse gelding owned by a client I'll call "Mary." Mary claimed Peter was "a little off—a little short." Watching Peter trot on the grass beside the barn, I could see no unevenness whatsoever, so we took him over to the blacktop driveway. Peter still trotted absolutely sound to my eye. This was only my second visit since Mary had moved with her six horses to her new 5-acre farm in my hometown, and the first time I had ever seen Peter trot. Mary had owned and ridden Peter for years, and she insisted he wasn't right, just "a little short."

I decided to do a lower leg flexion test, without even knowing which leg to start on. There was no apparent swelling or tenderness when I flexed Peter's left front pastern and fetlock, but when he trotted off after 45 seconds, he was obviously lame in the opposite leg. Feeling better that at least I could now see some lameness, I checked Peter's right front leg for any swelling or tenderness. Finding none, I repeated the lower leg flexion test on the right front side. After 45 seconds, Peter trotted off lame on his left front leg! I was just five years out of vet school, and I had never before seen opposite responses to hard flexion. I had not at all suspected laminitis, so it seemed like it took me about 20 minutes using hoof testers, checking digital pulses, and failing to find any leg tenderness to figure out that Peter's problem was in both front feet. I next improvised my own new "flexion" test and merely held up a front foot for about 20 seconds without any hard flexion. This magnified the slight "lameness" Mary could see in the opposite foot, so that we could both see him limp. This worked on both sides.

About fifteen years later, Dr. Chris Pollitt released an excellent video (9) of his Australian hoof circulation studies in which he demonstrated that a horse bearing excessive weight on one foot "surprisingly" (his word on the video) interrupts the laminar circulation to that foot.

Back to Peter in 1979—I was now confident Peter had a very slight soreness in both front feet, which I was unable to see without holding up an opposite foot. Peter had just been shod two days earlier with plastic pads over silicone. His feet were well shaped, but extremely short for his size. Mary mentioned a previous diagnosis of navicular disease for Peter, which was the reason for shoes and pads on the retired horse. However, Peter stood absolutely normally with no tendency to point either front foot. My hoof testers found no tenderness in his heel or frog area, but both feet were tender, even through the pads and silicone at his toes. I could feel no heat in his feet, but I could find a digital pulse in both feet. I, personally, could never feel a normal digital pulse. Having relatively insensitive fingers, I have always considered any digital pulse I can feel to be evidence of inflammation and increased blood pressure to the feet. In most horses with laminitis, I can feel the digital pulse in the front feet, but not the hind feet. When I can also feel it in the hind feet, I consider the horse to have laminitis in all four feet.

After about 20 minutes of examining Peter, I announced to Mary that he had the mildest case of acute laminitis that I had ever been called to examine (still true 35 years later). While I normally remove the shoes when I diagnose laminitis, because Peter's feet were so short, and he was freshly shod, and the laminitis was so mild, I decided he would be sorer if I removed his shoes. I simply gave Peter 10 cc of Bute IV. He was not the least bit overweight and was fed only a literal small handful of grain and two flakes of grass hay three times a day. He was kept in a very nice barn, in a stall with rubber mats, and just a little pine shavings to soak up the urine. Peter was turned out daily in a clean sand round pen with no pasture or weeds for him to eat. I had no explanation for why Peter had laminitis, but told Mary not to worry, because it was so mild, and there was no feed issue. This was 20 years before the Cushing's craze, but Peter showed no signs of Cushing's disease either.

Three days later, Mary called back to say that Peter had been fine for two days but was now moving "short" again. I still couldn't see any lameness, but this time it took maybe five minutes to repeat my exam with my hoof testers, hold up each front leg to watch him trot lame on the leg he had to stand on, and feel the digital pulse again. I repeated my mild laminitis diagnosis. Without my "flexion" tests on the driveway, Peter still looked absolutely sound to me, but short to Mary. I repeated the 10 cc of Bute IV, but still had no answer for Mary, other than possibly the extremely short feet, as to why her horse had laminitis, no matter how slight. I expected his feet would be better with a few more days of new growth.

On June 11$^{th}$, Mary called for the third time in seven days. Peter was no worse, and my opinion did not change, but after giving Peter 10 cc of Bute IV for the third time in a week to treat the very mild inflammation still in his feet, I sensed Mary's growing frustration with her new vet and suggested a second opinion at the Illinois Equine Clinic. They had diagnosed Peter's navicular disease several years earlier, but I didn't believe it had anything to do with the current problem.

Mary had Peter at the clinic that same afternoon. Unfortunately, the 10 cc of Bute I had given Peter that morning surely masked the mild laminitis I was seeing. Dr. Tom Phillips, the most respected equine referral veterinarian in the Midwest and a wonderful personal mentor for over 30 years, and his long-time partner, Dr. Joe Foerner, a past president of the American College of Veterinary Surgeons, put Peter through their usual meticulous lameness exam, including removing the shoes, multiple flexion tests, nerve blocks, and complete radiographs. Their conclusion was that Peter (and his X-rays) showed no sign whatsoever of laminitis on June 11th, but his old navicular disease was the cause of the persistent mild "lameness." Peter was de-nerved behind the pasterns the next day.

On June 22nd, after 10 days of stall confinement, Mary called me to remove Peter's sutures. When I arrived, a new farrier, Jim Powell, had just finished putting shoes and pads back on Peter, whom he had just met for the first time. The first thing the farrier said to me was, "this horse has been foundered!" This was 17 days after Mary had first called me because he was "off." I was grateful that someone finally agreed with me, but Peter was now sound (de-nerved), again freshly shod when I arrived, and there was still no feed issue to discuss. Peter looked and felt great. I was embarrassed by being overruled by the more experienced vets, but I did not feel I should ask Jim to remove a shoe to show me what he had just seen, and still did not search for a cause of the "founder."

The next sign of trouble was July 11th, 36 days after Mary had first called me. Peter was down in his stall and could not get up. His de-nerved feet hurt like crazy. I removed his shoes and pads while he was lying down, and both coffin bones had dropped through his soles overnight, after 36 days of untreated acute laminitis. After we put Peter to sleep without asking him to get up, a very distraught Mary mentioned that she had seen Peter eating leaves off an oak tree which hung over his round pen. When on a strict diet, horses will often eat what a horse with unlimited hay or pasture would never eat. Even a very mild toxin like oak leaves can kill a horse given enough time. I had never examined Peter's round pen area, but I have since traced a couple dozen other laminitis cases to horses eating leaves from trees and weeds. A couple walnut trees and one other oak tree have caused very mild laminitis. About a dozen cherry trees, and at least ten other times deadly nightshade eaten in overgrown fence lines, have triggered much more severe laminitis. The excessive stall confinement, shoes with pads, and very short feet probably also contributed to the inflammation, edema, and poor circulation in Peter's feet. De-nerving made Peter unable to give any further clues before he went down.

Ten years later, in July 1989 the late Dr. Jerry Peck, a special personal friend and mentor, called to chat. Dr. Peck, a past president of the American Animal Hospital Association, was the finest small animal veterinarian I ever knew, but his lifelong passion was racing trotting horses. After chatting awhile, Dr. Peck mentioned that one of his trotters, Talcott Jet, a 5-year-old stallion, was at a training farm north of Barrington where there was both a track and a swimming pool. Dr. Peck's trainer at Sportsman Park had felt Jet was a little sore all around, and he felt the pool might ease whatever ailed him since his vet at the racetrack could not pinpoint the soreness.

Dr. Peck would never let me pay him for taking care of my cats and dogs, but he occasionally asked me to help him with his horses, which I was honored to do at no charge. As clients who think they have a minor problem frequently say, Dr. Peck insisted that I not make a special trip to examine Talcott Jet, but he just asked if "the next time I was at the farm" I might "take a look at Jet."

About four days later, I was at the training farm for another client, and just before leaving, I asked the farm manager about Talcott Jet. The stallion just happened to be on the track training at that moment. The manager told me, "He comes out of the stall a little sore each morning but gets much better when he loosens up." He looked very normal as I watched him trot past a couple laps on the track. The manager felt the swimming pool should help his "generally mild early morning soreness." I agreed and left the farm without waiting to examine Jet. I did not report my casual observation to Dr. Peck.

Several months later I saw Dr. Peck and asked how Talcott Jet was doing. I was absolutely shocked to hear he had foundered badly and been put to sleep.

He had only been at the swimming pool farm two weeks before Dr. Peck had decided to take him home and turn him out in his backyard paddock to let some green grass and sunshine treat his nonspecific "muscle soreness." Dr. Peck personally fed and cared for him twice daily at home, but when the farrier came to reset his shoes about four weeks later, he found a widely separated white line and fully dropped soles. His feet were ruined before anyone realized he had laminitis for over six weeks.

In retrospect, Talcott Jet had been on extremely green and pure alfalfa hay along with full grain at both the racetrack and the swimming pool farm. Unlike many horses who founder, he was actually a bit of a hard keeper who required large amounts of grain and very good hay to maintain his weight when working. The soreness coming out of the stall each morning was his only visible sign of acute laminitis, which would get better as soon as he started getting fresh blood into his mildly inflamed feet. He was out all day at Dr. Peck's home, but while the hay was not as rich, he was on green grass and full grain to maintain his weight during the summer fly season. His laminitis was never recognized and treated.

Some may say these were both mild cases and have little in common with the severe cases too often seen in hospitals and on breeding farms. But the difference is only in degree, not in kind. You may only have a day or two to get it right with severe acute laminitis, but mild acute laminitis can linger a week or more before it is recognized, even by very experienced veterinarians. Horses never skip the acute stage. It is simply harder to notice in either a horse kept in a stall 24 hours with other ongoing lameness issues, or in horses at pasture 24 hours a day. Mild acute laminitis can be caught very early in horses ridden daily by sensitive riders. Since both front feet are likely to hurt equally, the horse won't nod or pound with one foot, but a good rider can easily feel the horse's reluctance to reach out as boldly as he normally would. These two horses were the hardest lessons I ever had to learn about laminitis. Laminitis must be recognized and correctly treated in the acute stage.

## AUTHOR'S CLARIFICATION OF THE LESSONS FROM THE DEATH OF PETER AND JET

I do NOT blame any of the three outstanding veterinarians named in this chapter for the deaths of Peter and Jet. My mistakes caused their deaths. These are mistakes that field veterinarians (and horse owners) make very commonly and lead to acute laminitis becoming chronic laminitis and founder before the disease is recognized.

Peter's acute laminitis was so mild that most owners would not have recognized it. It was invisible to me watching the horse trot. Only at the owner's insistence did I find it. I felt it was so mild that I did not worry when there were no obvious reasons for him to have it (other than extremely short shoeing, which might have added to the very mild inflammation from the oak leaves). I am the one who did not find the oak tree hanging over his round pen. Dr. Phillips and Dr. Foerner examined the horse at their hospital after I had given him 10 cc of Bute that morning, masking any mild inflammation in his feet. I should have asked the second farrier to remove the shoes he had just put on so I could also see the evidence of founder 10 days after his surgery. Peter's death was my fault.

Dr. Peck was a truly outstanding small animal veterinarian and trotting racehorses were his lifelong hobby. He never saw all the different versions of laminitis that I saw on so many different farms over the years. Laminitis is fairly rare in young horses in racing condition with almost no fat. Arthritis and muscle soreness are very common in young racehorses. Talcott Jet probably had acute laminitis at the racetrack. It was not recognized there by his trainer, by Dr. Peck, and probably also by the vet they used at the racetrack. The muscle soreness Jet showed was likely due to altering his gait to avoid pressure on his inflamed sore front feet. That is why he was sent to the farm with the swimming pool.

Dr. Peck did not want me to make a special trip because he knew I would not charge him to look at his horse. When I did see his horse a few days later he was trotting around the track quite nicely. Rather than wait to examine Jet, I merely watched and discussed him with the farm manager. Even if I had waited, I probably would not have seen any evidence of the laminitis after his workout. He reportedly only showed it when he first came out of his stall in the morning. But it was enough to kill him.

I am very skeptical when I hear veterinarians say that some horses do not go through the acute stage of laminitis, and founder overnight without anyone missing anything. Many of the stories in this book will help you recognize and respect laminitis when it can be fully cured!

# ~SECTION III~

## "PEAL" Cases, Pasture Endocrinopathy Associated Laminitis

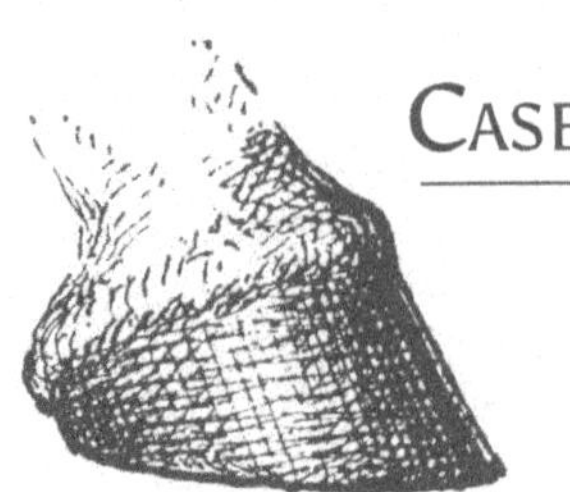

## Case Study

# "Easy Keepers"

## *Metabolic Syndrome, Insulin Resistant, Cushing's Disease, or Now—PEAL Horses*

THE STORIES IN THIS SECTION have been the most difficult for me to write, because the owner's role is so especially critical to the lifetime management and outcome of this type of horse. These stories are representative of at least 50 of my laminitis cases. Researchers, in their most recent effort to raise another $1 million for laminitis research, now call these "PEAL" horses, for Pasture and Endocrinopathy Associated Laminitis (28). I prefer to use the traditional horseman's term of "easy keepers."

These stories are not composites. Everyone is written from the medical records from each individual horse. All the names have been changed, so that I do not violate medical privacy. Most of the horses lived at home and the owners were the daily caretakers of the horses. The owner's competence, compliance, and confidence in my advice absolutely was the deciding factor in which of these particular horses lived long, drug free, useful lives versus which horses were euthanized within a year after following conflicting treatment advice from other sources.

If the horse owner does not believe the treatment rationale, it will not work. There are still many different theories used for treating laminitis (vasoconstriction, metabolic, endotoxic, diet, therapeutic shoeing, etc.) and some work much better than others. Unfortunately, because there is no single drug to test, traditional double-blind studies are not possible. Even withholding treatment and using placebos for the sake of science is inhumane and unethical with laminitis. For 42 years I have treated laminitis cases, including flare-ups of chronic laminitis, as a vasocompression, not a vasoconstriction problem. I have yet to see a case of laminitis progress "due to the mysterious nature of the disease."

University professors would have advocated blood tests for each of the horses in this section to determine whether they should be classified as Metabolic Syndrome, Insulin Resistant, Cushing's disease, or, most recently, "PEAL" horses. I prefer to use my clients' money for treatment rather than testing for an obvious diagnosis. "If it looks like a duck, walks like a duck, and quacks like a duck, it's probably a duck." I don't need a blood test to tell me it's a duck.

The dose for the dexamethazone suppression test to diagnose Cushing's disease is 20 mg. I have never given any horse that much dexamethazone at one time. I have seen at least three nasty cases of laminitis triggered by 5 to 10 mg of dexamethazone given to horses at high risk of laminitis. I have never blood tested any PEAL horses, because it would not have changed my diagnosis, treatment, or advice. Classifying the horse is not nearly as important as recognizing and treating the acute laminitis flare-ups.

Horses in this group require strictly limited diets, and absolutely do best with grass hays and grazing muzzles. Grazing muzzles were not yet widely used ten to twenty years ago, when most of these horses in this section first developed their periodic chronic laminitis.

## Case Study

# "Stepper"

### *20 years of successful vasocompression treatments after 7 Years of mostly unsuccessful vasoconstriction treatments*

STEPPER WAS A TENNESSEE WALKING Horse gelding who had been owned by Ted since he was purchased as a 4-year-old in 1987. Despite at least 20 flare-ups of chronic laminitis, Stepper would remain a favorite trail horse 30 years later. Stepper had experienced chronic laminitis symptoms for at least five years when I became his vet in 1994. Ted called me for a second opinion because his prior treatments of stall rest, therapeutic shoes, vasodilators, and pergolide from age five to ten seemed to be getting less effective, steadily more expensive, and more prolonged. By age 11, Stepper was lame much more often than he was sound.

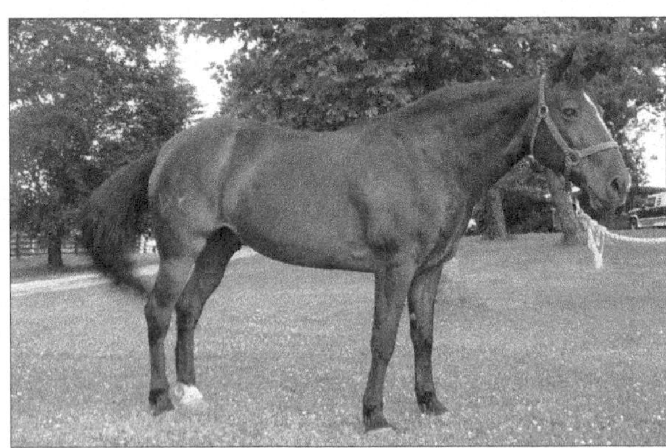

*Stepper*

Stepper had an enormous crest to his neck when I first saw him. He had dropped soles and a badly separated white line from five years of chronic laminitis. According to my records, he had "Grade III laminitis" that day with a "very easily detectable pulse in all four feet." I showed Ted how to monitor the digital pulse and explained my vasocompression theory of laminitis. Stepper had been prescribed Bute before, sometimes Banamine, often acepromazine or isoxsuprine and most recently, lifetime pergolide. The idea of a "minimum effective daily dose of Bute," which he was to adjust as necessary, was news to Ted. No one had explained the importance of the digital pulse or shown him how to monitor it.

Within a week Ted called to report that Stepper's digital pulse would be stronger in the stall first thing in the morning, but much softer after walking around the pasture in the afternoon. I explained how walking improves the circulation to the feet, and that it would be better if Stepper did not spend the night locked in a stall. With four horses on the eight-acre suburban farm, Stepper continued to be stall confined most nights for a few more years. Eventually, Ted realized that having Stepper out in the large lean-to at night decreased the frequency and duration of his periodic laminitis flare-ups.

In the 1990s, I was called to see Stepper for laminitis two or three times every year. Sometimes the cause was too much alfalfa in the "mixed hay." Once it resulted from a strictly grass hay which had been cut after the grass had gone to seed, effectively adding fine grain to the hay. Other times when the four horses had eaten the pasture down, there would still be wide areas of very short clover in the pasture. Clover does not need to be even 2" tall to sprout leaves. Any clover, alfalfa, or grain would absolutely set off Stepper's laminitis like a kid with a peanut allergy. Stepper had flare-ups several times when Ted was out of town for a few days, and his son or wife was feeding the four horses.

Nevertheless, over 19 years we treated Stepper for at least 20 flare-ups without further damage to his feet. In fact, his feet were far better now, after about twenty additional flare-ups that were quickly and properly treated, than they were in 1994! Stepper naturally had very tough hooves and he remained barefoot after I became his vet. Initially, the conventional farriers wanted to trim him like they were preparing the foot for a shoe, but would then leave him barefoot and watch him get more sore right after the trim. I would always ask Ted to have them trim the toe back from the front, not from the bottom, and lower the heels to get more frog pressure and realign the rotated coffin bones with the ground. I frequently trimmed his front feet myself because some of the conventional farriers had such difficulty understanding the concept. Ted then trimmed Stepper himself for a number of years, until natural trimmers moved to the area.

Stepper was not fed grain for about 18 years. At age 31, his molars were about worn out, and he was getting a scoop of Senior feed with beet pulp and finely chopped dehydrated hay blocks. He wore a muzzle most of the time when the pastures were growing. His crest was about half the size it was when he was younger. He was still an excellent and regularly used trail horse, especially for younger riders. Ted checked his digital pulse any time he walked with any hesitation. Stepper probably got a gram or two of Bute for a few days two or three times a year from age 25 to 30. When he was younger and fatter he needed close to 100 grams of Bute some years because of the extra weight he used to carry despite his diets. Ted never overfed him, but his "easy keeper" metabolism kept the weight on, and his hypersensitivity to alfalfa, clover, and grain would set off the laminitis.

A sad, but educational side note to Stepper's laminitis story is that six years after Ted called me for that second opinion, one of my favorite clients called Ted's prior vet for a second opinion on her horse Peanut, which I had just started treating for laminitis. Basically, the two owners traded vets. The patient I lost was just a three-year-old gelding whom I had cared for since his birth. The colt was born very small compared to his sire and dam. The owner always fed him more than he needed in the hopes it would help him get a little taller during the years he should have been growing. Instead, the extra feed just made him a very pudgy baby who was still much shorter than she had hoped he would be.

On March 1st, as a 3-year-old, he developed fairly mild Grade II laminitis. I could easily pick up either front foot, but after holding up either front foot for a minute, he would be very lame on the opposite foot walking on the concrete driveway. My records show he had an increased digital pulse pressure.

Despite still being short and pudgy, Peanut was being fed grain, alfalfa hay at night, and the clover was turning green very early that year in the pasture. I explained my laminitis treatment to the owner, prescribed 2 grams of Bute, asked her to stop the grain, get some grass hay, and use a muzzle to keep him off the clover. The owner called me to see him just two more times the following week. And while he was much better on the Bute, Peanut did not hurt enough yet for her to accept my feeding requests.

This owner was a wonderful longtime client and very intelligent. I could tell she was skeptical of my diagnosis, explanation, and requests. When I saw the colt twice more that week, he was not responding as quickly as I would have liked due to her reluctance to cut back on his calories and his turnout on a very hard dry lot. I asked her to diaper his feet to allow him to walk more comfortably with less Bute. When I did not hear from my client for about three weeks, I stopped by her small farm on my own. It had been raining and Peanut was full of himself jumping, running, and playing in the softer wet sand. His diapers were torn up, so I removed them to examine his soles. I left her a note thanking her for not shoeing him as had been her prior understanding for horses with laminitis. I also left her Dr. Pollitt's video (6) on hoof circulation to demonstrate the harmful effect of shoes on laminitis circulation.

My last note in his record was when I made a second courtesy visit on April 4th. He was "doing much better," with "bursts of jumping and tearing around the paddock." The owner had ridden him 10 minutes at a walk the previous weekend. He was still on Bute, and I asked her not to ride him until he was off Bute and sound. I asked her to keep his toes trimmed square, his heels low, and allow the quarters to grow enough to keep pressure off the sole.

When I did not hear from her again the next month, I stopped by uninvited a third time to find no one home, but my little patient had "therapeutic" shoes on. I never saw him or the owner again. I spoke to her on the phone, and she said she had chosen to follow other vet's advice on laminitis when mine "wasn't working," She never did accept my feeding advice.

Years later, I asked the other vet, a friend of mine for 30 years, how the colt did under his care. Sadly, the horse was sore his whole life, and he had to be euthanized at age 14 due to severe chronic laminitis. The therapeutic shoes, Banamine, stall rest, acepromazine, isoxsuprine, pergolide, and whatever else they tried did not help him as much as a reasonable diet and avoiding clover would have. If she had accepted my diagnosis, explanation, treatment, and management, he would never have suffered such a painful and short life. Luck had nothing to do with it. Laminitis is not a mysterious disease. It is simply misunderstood and mistreated by too many equine veterinarians.

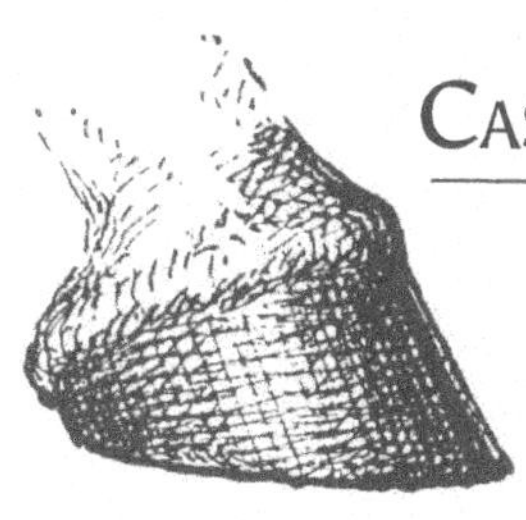

## Case Study

# "Traveler"

### *Five Flare Ups of Acute Laminitis at Age 10, Followed by 15 Nearly Perfect Years*

TRAVELER WAS A BLACK ARABIAN gelding that Karla purchased as a weanling. Traveler was the first horse for this very successful corporate executive who loved and treated her dogs and horses like children.

I met Karla and Traveler in September 1993, when he was the only weanling at a totally inappropriate boarding stable for older riding horses. He was there for one day when Karla recognized this was not a fit at all. Traveler needed to be on a farm where he could run, play, and grow up free with other horses. She had just purchased him from out of state, and quickly agreed to send him to my small farm until she could get a barn approved and built on her own wooded five-acre home site.

Karla previously met me when she called me about a stray dog that someone thought I might recognize. (I did not, and Karla kept the dog.) This turned out to be a four-year planning, permitting, and building process, during which I got to know Traveler, Karla, and her husband quite well as Karla visited Traveler nearly every day his first four years growing up on our small farm.

After Traveler eventually moved home, I continued to see him regularly for semi-annual shots and any minor cough or scratch.

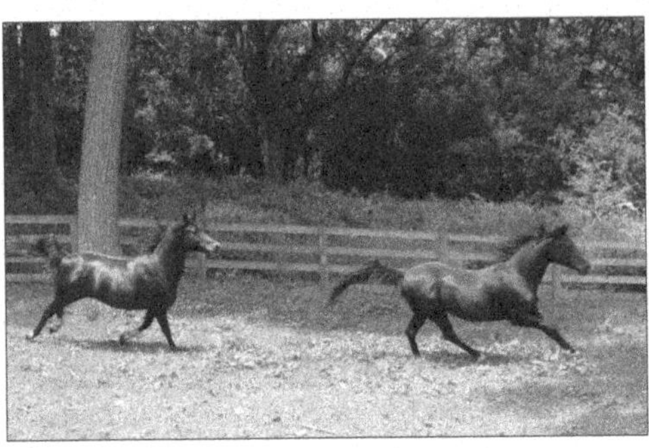

*Traveler (right)*

When Karla noticed the then 10-year-old Traveler moving just a bit hesitantly the week between Christmas and New Year's Eve 2002, she attributed it to the frozen ground and recent hoof trimming. Traveler's hooves were always on the brittle side, and Karla's very competent husband had purchased a complete set of hoof trimming tools for their two backyard Arabs. This allowed for more frequent rasping to keep the chronic wall chipping under control.

By New Year's Eve, Traveler was lying down in the pasture which was unusual, and it was apparent to Karla that she should call me to check Traveler's lingering and worsening sore feet. Unfortunately, she had no prior experience with laminitis and no reason to suspect it was an emergency. She was far too shy and polite to call me on a holiday weekend for what she assumed was a minor problem. When she did call me on January 2nd, I suspected laminitis from her description over the phone and saw Traveler that same morning.

He had Grade II acute laminitis (probably for at least a week between Christmas and New Year's) with an increased digital pulse pressure in both front feet. According to my records, he "walked hesitantly and avoided trotting," even in the snowy pasture. The icy ground around the barn was especially difficult, and the snow and ice packed in his feet added to his discomfort.

Even under his thick winter coat it was obvious to me Traveler had gained at least 40 pounds since I had seen him a couple months earlier. His mixed hay was about 60% high quality alfalfa. I administered Traveler both IV and oral Bute so I could trim his feet, lowering his heels and squaring the toes. I then wrapped both front feet with iodine/Epsom salts in the diapers and duct tape to cushion the icy ground and prevent ice balls from packing in the soles. I asked Karla to shake out the alfalfa from the hay and not give him that or grain—only grass hay and the minimum effective dose of Bute (1-2 grams of paste per day) to keep him moving comfortably and the digital pulse undetectable.

I rechecked Traveler two days later to change his diapers and again rasp his heels and toes. According to my records, he was "about 50% better, responding well, and he had already lost 10 pounds in just two days on grass hay!" On my next visit January 8th, Karla had some egg crate foam that we put inside the diapers, which helped him move even better. However, he still had an increased digital pulse pressure, so we continued the Bute paste as needed.

My next visit was ten days later whereupon Traveler was trotting and even cantering in the pasture with "minimal urging." He still needed his feet wrapped due to the frozen ground around the barn and his brittle hoof walls that caused more sole pressure than I liked. He was on 1 gram of Bute most days, skipping an occasional day to see if he was as comfortable without the medication.

After those three visits, I did not have to see Traveler again until April 28th. He had reportedly been off Bute and fine for over three months. He ran sound in his pasture for me on April 28th, but he trotted tender footed. I could feel an increased digital pulse pressure in all four feet. I was surprised Karla's husband was not trimming or rasping his feet as well as he should have, so I trimmed them myself that day and put him on what I thought would be another short course of Bute, while Karla watched his hay. He had fairly sparse pasture due to the heavy shade of many large oak trees. His paddocks had literally been cut out of an old forest.

Again, Karla had the laminitis quickly under control and I did not see Traveler again until June 13 and 14 when he was "still too fat" and had a "lump of sole putting uneven pressure on his left front sole," according to my records. I was again disappointed with the care his feet were getting from Karla's husband (who was never present for my visits) and despite my concerns, Karla defended her husband's efforts. But Traveler seemed fine running and playing in the pasture without Bute for another month before I visited him again July

9th. Traveler had been "running and playing the day before," but he now had clear serum oozing out of the white line at each side of the toe. This was the first evidence that he had some coffin bone movement since the start of his periodic laminitis more than six months earlier. I cleaned and trimmed the toes and put him back in diapers, that Karla continued to change daily.

Traveler was "much better" on my visit the next day, and by the 14th of July the laminitis seemed to be gone again. But the broken hoof wall was much worse on the right front. Through all these visits, I never saw Karla's husband who was supposed to be periodically rasping Traveler's feet. When I saw Traveler again on July 25 for another abscess, I was annoyed with Karla (the only time in over 20 years as a client and friend), because I felt she was letting the laminitis linger far too long. She was listening to every bit of advice I gave her, but I didn't understand why she or her husband were not adhering to my advice.

I had to see Traveler four more times the next two weeks for what I considered minor maintenance. By August 11, he was again "off Bute, running and trotting sound, and his feet were looking very good." Karla had started him on Farrier's Formula on her own about a month earlier. Karla kept his feet bandaged, rode him in the pasture, and on August 18th his feet looked even better. His substantial fever ring from that last week in December (when he was not treated the first week with acute laminitis) was by then 3⁄4" from the ground at the toe. After 7 1⁄2 months it still was not quite grown all the way out. On my August 25 weekly recheck he trotted a little short the first 20 to 30 seconds, then quite well. I rated him a "Grade 0.5 lingering laminitis" that day and prescribed 1 gram Bute every other day.

On September 4, he again had a detectable pulse in his left front leg after a week with no Bute. His abscess excavations at the toe were growing out nicely. A search of his paddock that day turned up a very small amount of nightshade growing through a back fence line which Traveler had eaten, as evidenced by the chew marks on the stalks. By September 12th, Traveler had again been off Bute for three days and was "full of himself," running hard, cutting and turning in the pasture without a hint of hesitation. On September 19th, he still looked 100% sound and sharp. I saw Traveler six more times the last three months of

2003 and his feet looked better and better each time I saw him until the end of his life at age 24, unrelated to laminitis.

This had been what I considered a very long, drawn out, recovery from simple acute laminitis since January 1st, with several very annoying relapses. I thought I knew Karla and her husband quite well from Traveler's four years at our farm, but Karla finally told me she had a heart attack in March 2003 when she found out about her husband's affair at work, and they were in the middle of a messy divorce. None of this helped Traveler's feet recover, although she did bandage his feet every other day. If I had known of her lack of support at home, I would have been more patient and helpful. The very good news is that Traveler did not have one single relapse of laminitis. His feet always looked excellent. He had been on Farrier's Formula every day for 11 years.

Traveler held his weight very well without any grain, alfalfa, or clover until he was 19 years old. By then his metabolism had changed and he was now able to eat small amounts of what he could not eat at all for about ten years. Karla absolutely trusted and followed my advice to the best of her ability. She now uses a "Natural Hoof Trimmer," and with Farrier's Formula 2X, Traveler had far better hooves than before his year of on/off laminitis started. Even the separated white line and dropped soles disappeared!

During his final fourteen years, he only had one brief flare up of laminitis when he found a few nightshade weeds that had grown in the heavily shaded fence line. A few days of Bute and pulling the three or four plants he was eating quickly returned him to full soundness with excellent feet. Karla did not believe he would eat nightshade since he had good pasture, until I held a stalk in front of his face and he went to grab it. You can note from his picture that he was fully recovered and never showed any sign of soreness after he was properly treated.

## Case Study

# "Cochise"

### *Zero Clinical Damage from 5-10 Bouts of Acute Laminitis, then Dead Within a Year When Switching Vets for More Modern Treatment*

BOB AND BETTY WERE A very successful retired couple with two large excellent Western trail horses, kept in their immaculate backyard barn and pasture. Their entire operation was always first class. They had owned their horses for at least ten years before they retired and moved out to my area. The "his and hers" trail horses were extremely well cared for.

Bob's Cochise looked like a typical Quarter Horse, but he was actually a very large Morgan. He had very minimal white line separation from chronic laminitis treated by his prior vet, a 30-year friend of mine, who had been my first laminitis mentor before I even started vet school. He treated the disease in the 1960s very similarly to the way I have treated laminitis since my graduation in 1974.

Bob was always rightfully proud of the way he kept their horses, and it really aggravated him when Cochise would have another attack of laminitis, no matter how minor and easily resolved. My records show I treated Cochise for 6 different attacks of laminitis the five years I took care of him (from age 20 to 25). They were all quickly resolved within a week or two, with a total of ten visits for the six minor relapses, with no additional damage to his feet. While Cochise was a big Morgan, he was not fat or unusually cresty, and Bob and Betty were always careful not to give him too much feed.

I could usually trace each minor flare-up to hay that had more alfalfa or clover leaves than Bob knew he could eat safely. A couple times Betty let Cochise graze the lush, fertilized lawn next to the barn for 20 minutes instead of the normally safe 10 minutes.

Other than his tendency to get laminitis very easily, Cochise showed no other signs of Cushing's disease. I don't normally consider Cushing's to be a "disease," because it is so common in older horses. Cochise always looked far younger than his early 20s when he was my patient. He did not have any excessive hair growth or delayed shedding in the spring. His muscling and body condition were always excellent. Other than the occasional five-to-ten-day bouts of mild laminitis he was the picture of health.

The last time I was called to treat Cochise for another laminitis flare-up, Bob was frustrated and certain he had done absolutely nothing wrong. The hay was very safe grass, and Betty had not been grazing him on the lawn. Cochise was not at all fat, and he was on just a true handful of grain with some supplements that had not been changed all year. I walked the wooded pasture that day looking for nightshade he might have eaten through the fence. I did find one shrub very obviously eaten over the fence. It was actually a very short tree, but the horses had been eating the top off it over the fence for years to make it look like a shrub at first glance. Though I am certainly not an expert, the leaves looked to me like it was a variety of wild cherry. Bob admitted the horses had been pruning the "bush" over the fence for years, but was adamant that it was not a cherry tree. He took me to see another tree which we both agreed was an untouched wild cherry tree across the fence. Bob was in no mood to argue, and I had to "agree to disagree" on the variety of the tree the horses had been eating over the fence.

My records show Cochise was sore enough that he needed 3 grams of Bute that day (probably as high a dose as he ever needed) and I provided Bob and Betty a bottle of 100 count 1-gram Bute tablets. I did not hear from Bob and Betty the next couple weeks, so I stopped on my own to look at Cochise while driving by their farm. Cochise was "walking very well" according to my notes that day, but I saw that he had shoes on for the first time since I had known him. They were on backwards, a technique sometimes used by other vets to unload the toe for laminitis while slightly raising the heel. I also noticed that there was a tube of Banamine paste by Cochise's stall. They had obviously called another vet for a different opinion of the laminitis flare-ups. I happened to see Betty in town six months later. She said, "Oh, you were out of town the next time we called you, so we had Dr. X come, and he tested Cochise for Cushing's disease and put him on pergolide. That's why he kept getting laminitis." I heard from other clients that Cochise had to be put to sleep before another year passed. The Banamine, pergolide, and therapeutic shoes obviously did not work as well as identifying and eliminating the triggers and using the minimum effective daily dose of Bute had worked for Cochise's prior 15 years (including the previous 10 years my mentor had treated his occasional laminitis).

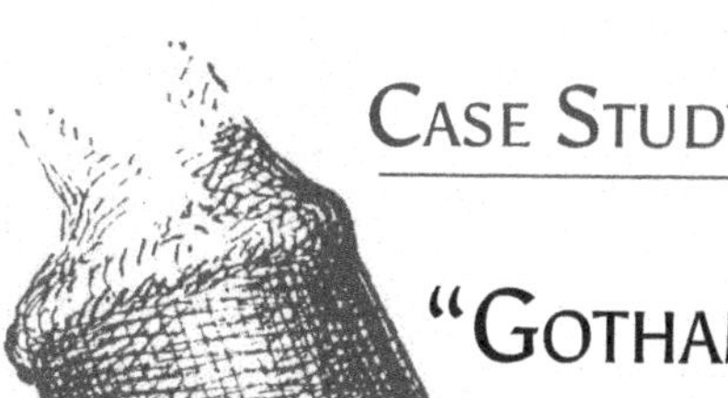

## Case Study

# "Gotham Gold" and "Hershey"

*Exceptions to the breed tendencies.*

DIFFERENT BREEDS OF HORSES DO have different traits and tendencies, but there are so many case studies included in this book because every horse must be treated as an individual, and there are many exceptions to the general rules. Two interesting horses which come to mind have feet opposite their breed tendencies. Hershey and Gotham Gold were regular patients for over 20 years. I knew them very well as individuals. Neither horse had ever had more than a hint of laminitis. Hershey came without papers, but she appeared to be a Morgan crossed with a small Quarter Horse. She was 30+ years old with tiny feet and was finally showing signs of her age. Gotham was a 25-year-old, off-the-track Thoroughbred with excellent feet who could pass for a 10-year-old! These were first horses for a retired couple in their 70s, who kept them at an excellent boarding stable and rode them three or four times most weeks for the past 20 years.

I remember Gotham's pre-purchase exam like it was yesterday. He was bought at Arlington Park by Cathy, the stable owner and trainer. She was reselling him at a modest profit to Barry who had been learning to ride on Cathy's lesson horses. Gotham had just started his retraining for trail use when Barry decided he would rather own than rent a horse. Gotham's five years at the racetrack had reduced his range of fetlock motion and caused traumatic arthritis of the fetlock. He had a medium response to flexion tests. He was not lame, but he was also not suitable for jumping or serious dressage, the two most common second careers of off-the-track Thoroughbreds.

Barry assured me that he was not interested in jumping or dressage. He was more interested in riding the adjacent forest preserve trails with his proudly preserved military saddle. He simply liked Gotham's size and personality. He was an impressive looking horse. Since Gotham's new level of work was to be so much easier than his racing years, I felt his arthritis could be managed. I would prefer 24-hour turnout for this horse, but he was scheduled for about four hours a day. Otherwise, the situation was excellent for the horse—and enough of a challenge for Barry.

Barry's wife had purchased Hershey a year earlier, but Gotham was far bigger and more spirited. Because Cathy was to be their resident trainer, I approved the purchase with Barry's understanding that Gotham, like buying a used car, was coming with pre-existing arthritis issues. Barry indeed successfully managed the arthritis with low levels of Bute and regular moderate exercise for nearly 20 years.

The only hint of laminitis these two horses had previously was when Hershey got sore footed a couple times because of the hard trails. Both horses were always shod and Hershey had very small narrow feet. Fortunately, she always had a small rider who rode her gently. Nevertheless, the constant shoeing did encourage her heels to become even more narrow, and this gave her a couple brief periods of foot soreness. It was not unlike road founder, but it came more from her heels than her toes and was quickly corrected by a very good farrier.

I was out of town three weeks when Hershey again became sore footed right after a trim, so a different vet was called. He correctly diagnosed acute laminitis with a detectable pulse in all four feet. He prescribed 3 grams Bute per day and strict stall rest. After a week, when Hershey was even more sore footed, despite the 3 grams per day of Bute, I was called for a second opinion on my patient of 20 years.

I could not get to the barn that same day before Barry and his wife had to be back home, but I knew the horse well. Hershey had been trimmed and left barefoot the day before the lameness started, so I asked Barry to get some diapers, put iodine and Epsom salts in them and wrap them on her front feet. Then, rather than stall confinement, I asked for her to have as much time as possible wandering the indoor arena.

When I saw Hershey the next day, they reported she was walking significantly better than she had walked in a week. I could only find a slight digital pulse in one front foot. She turned easily, and picked up either front foot easily. I asked them to immediately reduce the Bute. Cathy asked if she could go back on grass. I thought the grass (shared with about ten other horses) should be safe for her in mid-June, but when I saw the two grass pastures, there was a problem with each. One was eaten fairly short but filled with clover. The other was knee high and had gone to seed. Horses who ate the tops off that grass were getting very fresh grain! Both lush clover and a grass pasture gone to seed are dangerous to a horse recovering from laminitis, even if the cause was very thinly trimmed soles. The week of stall confinement prevented Hershey from getting the circulation she needed through her swollen laminae to heal her feet.

I called Barry three days later to ask how Hershey was doing. He answered, "She has never felt better in her life. She's dragging Georgie around when she takes her out to graze a little!" It had been 36 hours since her final single gram dose of Bute. I suggested that at her age, a half gram of Bute a day might be appropriate for her, but not 3 grams per day. Barry was 78 years old himself, and he readily agreed.

Hershey began a typical case of acute laminitis three weeks earlier, but stall confinement was not the best treatment for her. With the inflammation in her feet from the thin sole trim, and the clover and seed tops in her pastures, she had three reasons for acute laminitis. Most of all she needed walking on soft sand to treat the stagnant blood from stall confinement before the laminae started to fail.

Every horse and every case has unique aspects. But the protocol is the same: identify and remove the triggers and promote circulation to the hoofs.

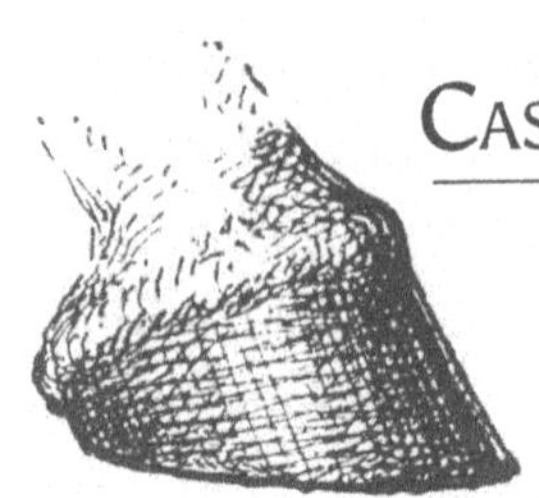

# Case Study

## "Bingo"

### *Severe, Acute, Grade IV Laminitis—"Miraculous Cure"—Then Lingers*

BINGO WAS AN 8-YEAR-OLD Paint gelding who had severe Grade IV acute laminitis Saturday, March 7, 2009. Since doing Bingo's very simple pre-purchase exam just six months earlier, I had seen Bingo five or six times for standard vaccinations, dental checks, and just in passing through his boarding stable. Coincidentally, I had also seen him just the day prior to his severe acute laminitis, thoroughly searching his mouth for a suspected bit problem. Each time I had seen Bingo, he had impressed me as a very solid, young, sound, and well-balanced "first horse" for a new family. Bingo always seemed to be easily kept near an ideal weight for his body type. He never struck me as being on the fat side or the thin side, and certainly not at risk for Grade IV acute laminitis.

Having just seen Bingo on Friday the 6th of March, I was very surprised to receive a call from his owner, Angie, the next day. Cathy, the stable owner/manager, had called her saying that Bingo "could not walk, was having trouble standing up, and that she needed to see if the vet could come to the barn right away." Neither Angie nor I had seen anything the day before suggesting colic, laminitis, or a neurologic problem. Cathy was a very experienced, longtime client with very good judgment, and I readily agreed to meet her at the stable by 4:00 that Saturday afternoon.

While driving to the stable, I speculated that it was most likely acute laminitis, which is just as much an emergency as colic. Some laminitis researchers (and professors, who believe everything researchers publish) claim that by the time lameness is seen, permanent damage has already been done to the laminae. I disagree. Microscopic damage may be visible on euthanized research horses in the developmental stage (prior to lameness) of experimentally induced acute laminitis, but I don't believe laminar edema in clinical cases needs to cause permanent damage in a properly and promptly treated horse, any more than a headache or hives should leave permanent damage. I know the length of the "window of opportunity" (equivalent to the "golden hour" in human heart attack, stroke, and brain injury victims) to cure acute laminitis without any clinical damage is directly related to the severity of the attack. Severe cases have a much shorter window, and they need to be treated correctly without delay. The longer laminitis is allowed to linger, the more likely there is to be permanent damage. A Monday appointment would have been disastrous for Bingo.

When I arrived, Bingo was standing in the back of his stall while all the other horses in the barn were up front eating dinner. He had to be dragged and pushed out of his stall. Turning to the left in the concrete aisle obviously hurt a great deal, as he took very short and painful steps. His digital pulses were throbbing behind both front fetlocks. They were softer, but also easily detectable in his rear fetlocks. I asked Angie, Cathy (who had a nearly identical case of sudden severe acute laminitis with her horse, Dots, eleven years earlier), and Jorge, the main caretaker, to each feel the throbbing digital pulses. I wanted each of them to use the decreasing strength of the digital pulse to help determine how much Bute to give on subsequent days, since I always try to give the minimum effective daily dose of Bute as the horse recovers.

Bingo hurt too much for me to even attempt to pick up a front foot, or even tap on his hooves with the hoof testers (I would not want a doctor tapping on my head after I told him I had a severe headache). I planned to start him on 12 cc of Bute IV for the pain and inflammation, and 6 cc of Lasix IM for the edema which was compressing the blood vessels in his sensitive laminae and creating the extremely painful oxygen deficit there. For maybe the only time in 42 years, I had no injectable Bute in my truck that Saturday afternoon. Instead, I used 3 grams of Bute paste because I believe oral medications require a little higher dose for the same effect as IV medications.

I then asked for Bingo to be walked and turned loose in the large indoor arena. Cathy asked if she could cold hose him in the wash rack on the way to the arena. I certainly agreed that would help remove some pain and inflammation while we were waiting for the drugs to work. When we got him to the arena after about five minutes of hosing, Bingo was already starting to walk better. After one slow lap around the arena, I asked the owner to turn him loose. He did not yet walk as freely as I had hoped. Obviously, the oral Bute paste was taking longer to reach effective blood levels than the IV Bute would have done immediately.

I asked Cathy for a companion horse from the stable who would also wander around the arena with the expectation that Bingo would follow him. Cathy runs one of the best managed stables in the Chicago suburbs, and she knew immediately what type horse I was asking for. I asked her to drop half a flake of grass hay in four or five different areas to encourage the two horses to walk from pile to pile. I stopped Cathy and asked her to first bring the hay back to the concrete aisle and shake out each flake in front of the stall door of a horse who could use a little extra feed.

Cathy and I shook out each flake of hay, picked the stems off the top and found an incredible amount of leaves and seeds left on the concrete floor. The hay field had been cut after it had gone to seed, so the leaves and seeds left on the floor amounted to several handfuls of very high protein, which I consider much more likely to trigger laminitis than starches or Non-Structural Carbohydrates.

In northern Illinois, I have seen about 20 times more cases of laminitis caused by clover and alfalfa hays than by grass hays. With clover and alfalfa, the leafier the hay, the higher the protein, the more likely it is to cause laminitis. Shaking huge piles of leaves out of these hays can make them much safer to feed horses at risk for laminitis.

About 20 minutes after receiving the Lasix, Bingo stretched out to urinate a substantial volume. This indicated to me that the Lasix was drawing water out of his tissues, especially the edematous laminae in his feet. He was significantly more comfortable when I left. Cathy and Angie watched him wander with the other horse until 10:00 pm, and when they left both horses were comfortable in the large arena.

Angie spent the rest of the night reading the good, the bad, and the ugly about laminitis on the internet. There was no shortage of conflicting advice and many stories of months of agony-unlike the 15 minutes she had witnessed in her horse.

Cathy and Angie called me separately Sunday morning to tell me that Bingo was walking normally and even trotting easily. Cathy felt it was quite exciting to literally watch a horse recover from such a serious disease before her eyes in one evening. Angie wanted to know if he could go back in his stall. It had been raining for three days and was still too cold and windy to be comfortable in a muddy paddock.

I told Angie, since other boarders would want to use the arena Sunday afternoon, he could certainly go back in his stall, but that she should provide no grain, shake the leaves and seeds out of his hay, give him 1 gram of Bute paste, and continue to check the strength of his digital pulse. Angie called back later that afternoon to report that Bingo had been lying in his stall much of the day Sunday. When they got him up to walk in the aisle, he walked quite normally, but they could still feel his pulse in his front fetlocks, but not in the rear. I told her that was an indication that the stall time had decreased the circulation to his now mildly inflamed laminae. Very mild laminitis which is either unrecognized or allowed to linger is much more likely to cause some permanent structural damage with either rotation or sinking of the coffin bone as the weakened laminae gradually lose their grip with less than optimum circulation.

I next saw Bingo and Angie on Tuesday, March 10th. He was doing quite well, but I was concerned that he still had a mild pulse in his front feet. I gave Angie a half dozen case histories I had written up similar to Bingo's to reassure her, since she had read of so many disasters on the Internet. As long as she continued to monitor him and treat with the minimum effective dose of Bute, I expected no problems.

Bingo spent the next four nights wandering the arena, but he was back in his stall most of each day. Angie asked me to come back and recheck Bingo on Thursday, March 12th, because although she could not feel his digital pulse when he came in from a night in the arena, she could feel the pulse behind his fetlock after a few hours in his stall, and he was still spending much of his stall time lying down. After five days he was still getting 1 or 2 grams of Bute a day. Because he had made such rapid improvement to 90% of normal the first night, Angie was wondering why the last 10% of recovery was lingering.

When I saw Bingo, on the sixth day of his acute laminitis attack, he walked out of his stall easily, but it was still easy for me to feel his digital pulse. There was a huge pile of "grass hay" in his stall. His stall card said, "NO GRAIN," but his hay ration had been increased to 4 large flakes morning and night to make up for stopping his grain.

I took out some of the hay and shook it over the concrete aisle. After then picking up the stems from the top, there was again a great pile of leaves and seeds on the floor. There was no need to increase his normal hay ration from 3 to 4 flakes twice a day, as Bingo was not at all thin. Although he had no arch to the crest of his neck, when I felt the top of his neck, it was surprisingly thicker and stiffer than I had assumed. Bingo hid his extra pounds very well. I always tell horse owners I like to be able to feel a few ribs, but not see them. I certainly could not see Bingo's ribs, nor could I feel even one rib. Bingo had appeared much more fit than when I actually felt his neck and chest.

I explained to Angie, Cathy, and Jorge that while Bingo was obviously greatly improved, he was not yet over the laminitis. His body fat was still storing and releasing some of the endotoxins that triggered the laminitis a week earlier. He did not need the extra flakes of too rich hay to replace the grain that was being withheld, and the amount of arena time versus stall time directly affected the need for continuing the low level of Bute. They readily understood how these factors (the fat, the feed, and the stall time) worked together, and everyone wanted him off Bute as soon as possible, while still making the arena available to the other boarders now that Bingo was not in imminent danger.

A new load of hay arrived that afternoon which did not have nearly as many seeds and leaves in it. Bingo spent several more nights in the arena, and he received his last dose of Bute on March 17, ten days after the severe attack had started.

The next time I happened to be at the stable for other horses was March 27th, and by coincidence, Angie was just saddling Bingo in the aisle for a lesson with Cathy. They had not felt a pulse in ten days. Angie had ridden Bingo several times, and he acted like nothing had ever happened. I briefly watched the lesson and Bingo, Angie, and Cathy all looked very happy. According to his farrier, Bingo had no visible damage from his one-day attack of Grade IV acute laminitis, which lingered nine more days as Grade I. He did not have another soreness of any type for the more than eight years I saw him.

# ~SECTION IV~

## Four Very Severe Cases that Fully Recovered

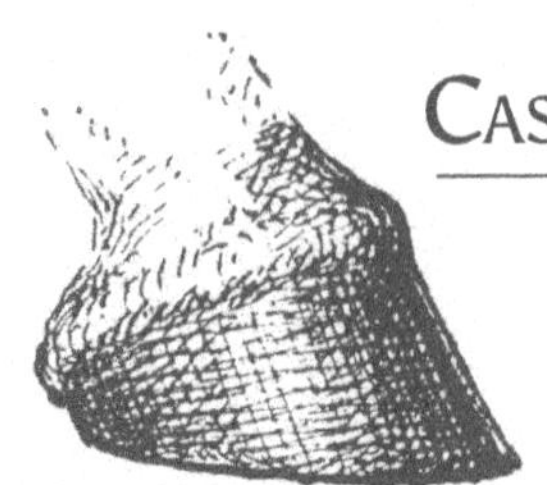

## Case Study

# "Raindrop"

*My First Ever Laminitis Case—*
*Choke Cherry Trees*
*(2 Years Before I Entered Vet School)*

IN AUGUST 1968, BEFORE I had even applied to veterinary school, I saw my very first case of acute laminitis, and an old fashioned, but very effective treatment. I was still fairly new to horses when Raindrop, a 3-year-old Spotted Saddlebred filly came down with sudden, severe laminitis. Raindrop and another young riding horse were being kept in a newly fenced off area of a racehorse farm. She and the other horse were being allowed to "eat down" the overgrowth prior to cleaning the new pasture for eventual use by the trotters and pacers on the farm. Raindrop was found one Saturday morning refusing to move in the pasture, so the vet was called. Dr. Walt Dalitsch arrived quickly and explained that the 3-year-old filly had severe acute laminitis—sudden inflammation in her feet. Since she was so young and not the slightest bit fat, he asked what she had been eating. She was being given a little grain, but mostly was being allowed to scavenge the scrub brush in the new pasture.

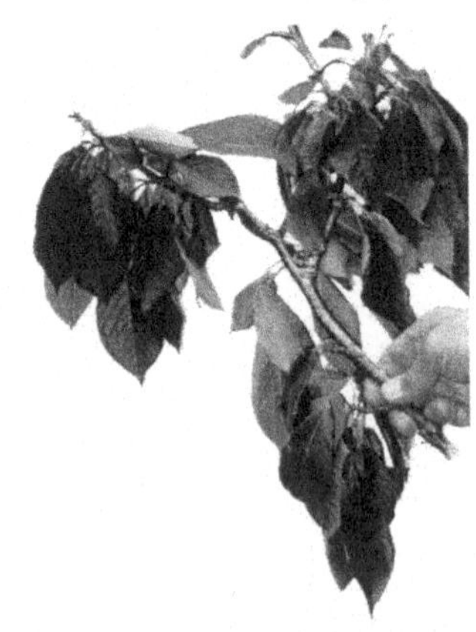

*Eaten Cherry Tree Leaves*

After giving the filly a shot of Bute, Dr. Dalitsch asked to see the pasture. We walked down the lane with him to inspect the area, and he quickly pointed out a young tree from which at least one of the two horses had been stripping the bark and tender leaves. He said it was a Choke Cherry whose bark and leaves are toxic to horses. Dr.

Dalitsch then gave Raindrop a gallon of mineral oil and told us since there was no creek on the farm, we should dig up and flood a corner of one of the clay floored stalls in the barn for Raindrop to stand in until the inflammation was out of her feet. He said her response depended on how quickly the oil helped clear the cherry tree toxins from her gut. He said the Bute was not so much for its pain killing effect, as for its anti-inflammatory effect on her feet. We would know she has recovered when she could walk out of the stall without pain and without drugs.

Dr. Dalitsch, who became my valued personal mentor for the next 45 years, was a relatively new graduate himself at that time. However, he was most fortunate to have learned his acute laminitis treatment from Dr. Bill Bauman, who had grown up with working draft horses on his dad's farm in the 1920s. Doc Bauman had gone to Iowa State University's Veterinary College in the 1930s. At that time tractors were replacing the majority of America's working draft horses as America struggled through the long Depression. The racehorse and pleasure horse industries were limited to only the very wealthy when Doc Bauman was in college. Very little was taught about horses in the vet schools in the 1930s because the professors thought the horses were all being replaced.

Of note, only nine of our current 30 U.S. vet schools were open during the long Depression of the 1930s. Doc Bauman graduated from vet school just five months before Pearl Harbor was attacked. As one of the very few veterinarians in northern Illinois, he was given an "essential services" deferment to stay home and treat farm animals during WWII. Doc Bauman's professors had very much ignored equine medicine, telling the students that the few farmers who still had horses would be replacing them very soon with tractors. Even the Army's remaining cavalry horses were of little use by 1942. No one had predicted the explosion of pleasure horses in the 1960s and '70s.

Just prior to the introduction of most modern pharmaceuticals, the 1942 *U.S. Department of Agriculture Yearbook* (19) still reported that acute laminitis was "one of the few ailments which may be improved by bleeding...." Dr. Dalitsch did not bleed Raindrop. Both Bute and Lasix were commonly used to reduce inflammation and edema by 1968, but the cold mud bath was a serious part of Raindrop's rapid recovery from such severe acute cherry tree laminitis as a three-year-old.

Raindrop had a couple much less dramatic flare-ups of pasture laminitis over the next five years that were also successfully treated by Dr. Dalitsch. When the Kellys moved to California in 1973, her feet still looked very good with virtually no damage from her attacks of laminitis in Illinois. Unfortunately, when I visited their California farm in 1979, after I graduated from vet school myself, Raindrop was badly foundered.

The farm in California fed mostly irrigated alfalfa and oat hay. Raindrop was kept outside 24/7, and I strongly suspect she continued to have frequent, milder, and likely unrecognized attacks of laminitis her first six years there. I also suspect the California vets whom the Kellys called frequently for their racehorses treated laminitis much differently in the '70s than Dr. Dalitsch and I did, or than we continue to treat it 45 years later.

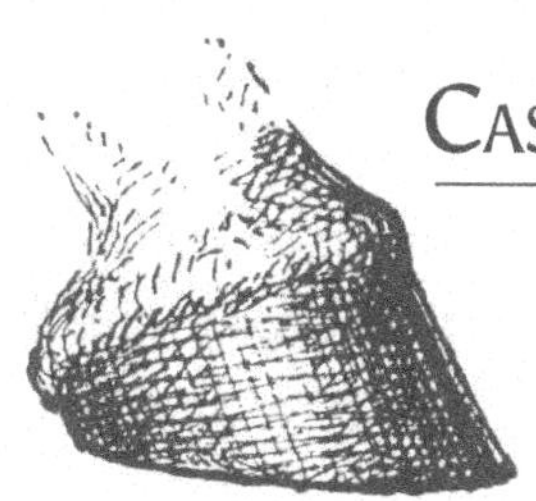

## Case Study

# "Dixie"

### *Extremely Painful Laminitis*

THIS IS ONE OF THE most severe and painful acute laminitis cases ever, but a perfect recovery with zero damage!

This case happened in 1982. It was two and a half years before I would hear the late, and truly great, Texas farrier, Burney Chapman, lecture the AAEP in Dallas (32) on his incredibly bloody anterior hoof wall resections. The removal of most of the hoof wall was followed by prolonged, extremely precise, and expensive heart bar shoe protocols for nine months (or maybe a lifetime) to arrest the constant pain of founder disasters. Immediately after that two-hour lecture, I asked Dr. Matthew MacKay-Smith, one of the country's most well-known veterinarians (as the medical editor of *EQUUS*), "If people can spend that much money, time, and effort to 'salvage' a badly foundered horse, why don't they just treat the inflammation and prevent the founder?"

I will never forget the answer I got from this man who was much smarter than I ever hope to be: "Son, there is no inflammation in laminitis. It is a vasoconstriction caused by an imbalance of rennin and angiotensin, produced by the kidneys to regulate blood pressure." I was aware of the kidneys' role in regulating systemic blood pressure, but I had believed, since I was a first-year vet student in 1970, that the vasoconstriction with laminitis was localized outside the hoof, as an attempt to overcome the vasocompression from inflammation within the hoof. Dr. Chris Pollitt's photos (7) proved the separate pastern vasoconstriction and laminar vasocompression locations conclusively to me. However, at the 1992 AAEP meeting in San Francisco, Dr. Pollitt used the same slides I saw in *EQUUS* to deny any inflammation was present in acute laminitis. It would be 2007 before I saw an explanation of oxygen sensors regulating localized blood pressure responses, which I had always believed were part of any animal's innate mechanism for homeostasis (27).

I had gone home from the 1984 AAEP Convention and started sending letters, articles, case reports, and opinion pieces to *EQUUS*, as I believed it was the best magazine directed at owners of all breeds of horses. The professional veterinary journals simply dismissed my case reports as insignificant "anecdotes." Dr. MacKay-Smith at least responded with his opposing views on laminitis, and he did eventually publish one very dramatic case report I submitted in the June 2000 issue of *EQUUS* ("Fame") (32). He never believed my theory of laminitis, and most of my prior and subsequent submissions were rejected with, "You've had your 15 minutes of air-time."

Cases like Dixie always reinforced my theory, both before and after I'd seen the proof in the research. This happened both before and after I realized the majority of vets believed the professors' and researchers' interpretations of the latest research finding of the year.

A very interesting 2009 survey completed by 592 AAEP members (33) ranked the equine diseases most in need of more research. Laminitis was the clear winner with 63% of the vets listing it at, or near the top of, their list. Most people interpreted that survey as justification to spend millions more on laminitis research. I on the other hand, ask why did 37% of the vets who filled out the survey not even mention laminitis, out of the dozen diseases reported? I had believed (from informal feedback from colleagues since that 1984 AAEP meeting) that between 1/4 and 1/3 of practicing vets treat laminitis very similarly to me, and similarly have very little problem with laminitis. According to this survey, it could be that 37% of vets did not mention laminitis, because they understood it is a very predictable disease, when the vet is called early and treats it correctly. Since hospital and university vets (who lose so many laminitis cases) were included in the survey, it may well be that over 50% of field vets have very little problem curing laminitis. Remember, laminitis always precedes founder, which is not fully curable.

In 1982, Dixie was a large, healthy, and very well fed Quarter Horse type mare. She was high strung with horrible ground manners. Dixie would break cross ties and halters at the slightest provocation. She spun her rear at any vet who dared enter her stall. Nevertheless, she was a good trail horse for her very mild-mannered young owner Rita, who displayed extreme patience with Dixie's lack of barn manners.

Rita and her sister, Mary Jo, lived and worked in Chicago, but they spent most of every weekend in the country with their two horses. It was a beautiful May Saturday afternoon when Rita realized that Dixie just was "not herself" on the trail. Normally she was sound, solid as a rock, and very eager on the trail, but this day she just seemed a bit reluctant and tender-footed all around. She had four of the most perfect feet I have ever seen on any horse. Rita dismounted and checked all four feet to see if Dixie had a stone stuck in her frog. Finding nothing and puzzled, Rita walked Dixie two miles back to her barn. Rita weighed barely 100 pounds, and it would have been fine with me if she had ridden the powerful mare back to the barn, but Rita always was careful, and too tolerant, with Dixie.

When Rita and her sister returned to the barn Sunday afternoon, Dixie refused to come out of her stall. They were used to Dixie being the boss, so they tried bribing her with feed and treats. She ate everything they offered but pinned her ears when they tried to lead her out of the stall. Neither of the girls had enough experience with horses to even suspect laminitis, but just before going home, they called me from the barn to check Dixie on Monday. Very fortunately, I was home that Sunday and answered my own phone.

A very brief description of Dixie's odd behavior told me that Monday would be way too late. I told Rita to wait for me, and I would be at the barn in 30 minutes. In the meantime, I asked her to get some help to get Dixie out of her stall and into the sand indoor arena. When I arrived, a couple cowboys had literally drug Dixie, with the aid of an aluminum scoop shovel, into the sand arena less than 100 feet from her stall. Dixie stood there dripping with sweat from the effort. All four legs were swollen to the knees and her hocks looked like stove pipes. For the only time in her life, she did not move a step as I examined her. She had a temperature of 104° F and a throbbing digital pulse in all four feet. I immediately gave her 12 cc of Bute IV and 10 cc of Lasix IV for the edema. We then brought out a hose and proceeded to make a muddy mess where she stood just inside the doorway of the indoor arena. I made sure both of the sisters felt the throbbing pulse, explained why it was so prominent, and told them they would have to use the strength of that pulse to gauge her need for Bute while she was recovering.

After about ten minutes of hosing all four feet with cold water, we were able to walk her a little in the soft sand. We returned to the wet sand and hosed all four feet and lower legs again. The next time we walked, she stretched out to urinate what seemed like a gallon. The Bute and cold water were controlling the pain in her feet enough to let her walk a little more each time. Within 30 minutes, I was able to hold up a front foot just long enough to get her shoes off. After another short walk I squared her toes and lowered her heels. She walked even better as fresh blood was now able to get through her severely swollen laminae.

As I was preparing to leave, Rita asked how long they should continue the hosing and light walking. I suggested all night would be best for Dixie. They readily agreed, and when I returned Monday morning, Dixie was about 90% better. She was back dancing around when I just went to check her digital pulse pressure. She walked readily on her own and her temperature was back to normal without any antibiotics. I had only given her 12 cc of Bute and 10cc of Lasix the day before. The hosing and walking barefoot in the sand had removed nearly all the visible swelling and edema. I simply gave another 10 cc of Bute and told the sisters to go home but leave Dixie loose in the sand arena with just grass hay and water.

When I rechecked Dixie on Tuesday, she was still just about 90% recovered. The stable wanted the arena back for other boarders, so the sisters roped off a small area between the two barns where the runoff of both roofs kept the area muddy that time of year. We switched Dixie to just 2 grams of Bute a day in a small handful of sweet feed, plenty of grass hay, and the girls used their hose to make some serious mud between the barns.

I did not see Dixie again for nearly a week. This mare who had always been so unpleasant for me to examine was a pathetic site after her week in "jail" between the barns. Her long tail dragged in the mud, and she constantly splattered herself when she went after the flies with her mud-loaded tail. When they brought her out for me, she pranced up and down the driveway without a hint of foot soreness. Dixie had naturally round, tough hooves, which helped her a great deal. We reduced Dixie to just 1 gram of Bute per day for almost a month. The girls would occasionally skip a day of Bute only to find a slight pulse again. They stopped the Bute when they could no longer find the pulse at her fetlock.

The cause of the severe laminitis was a failure to reduce Dixie's winter grain ration when the spring pasture came in with very lush rapid growth. It did not help that the stable owner was a feed dealer, and he liked people to see his fat horses. In the late 1980s, Dixie and I moved about ten miles in opposite directions. I never enjoyed working with her, so her owners eventually switched to the closer vet. I did, however, see her and Rita once every few years into Dixie's late 20s. She never had a second bout of laminitis. Her farrier never saw the slightest white line separation or flat sole.

This case is the extreme example that, contrary to what researchers frequently claim, there is no permanent clinical damage when the horse first shows pain from laminitis. If I had waited another 24 hours before seeing her, I am sure there would have been laminar damage or destruction.

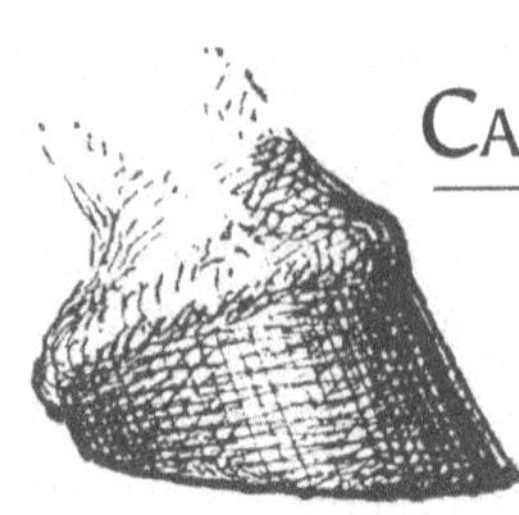

## Case Study

# "Killer"

### *Complete Cure Despite Poor Compliance*

BILLY CALLED AT 6:00 AM on an unusually hot May 15, 1992. He was caring for Killer, who was down in the pasture and wouldn't get up for his morning grain. The owner was one of my most peculiar clients, but the farm was less than two miles from our farm, so I told Billy to try to get him up to the barn, and I'd be over in a few minutes.

Killer was an eight-year-old ex-racehorse, too slow to hurt himself, and retired due to lack of interest. He would have made a nice project for a new career, but he and the farm were owned by an eccentric retired surgeon who had gone to law school in his 60s. His new business card now read, "Practice limited to Medical Malpractice." His second career was suing former colleagues from his first career!

The doctor/lawyer's wife, a nurse, was the one with the real interest and affinity for horses. Unfortunately, she had died a few years earlier, and the farm operation was now a shambles.

Billy was hired after doing time for some barroom brawls. It was his first job with horses, but he fed and watered about 25 assorted brood mares, foals, and retirees by himself. Not the best situation, but they always had plenty of feed and pasture. I learned later that day that they had run out of hay, so Billy fed the horses in this pasture double their normal grain!

When I arrived, Billy had Killer literally halfway in the barn door. He wouldn't go any further. He was bloated and sweating with cherry red gums. Obviously numb with colic pain, I immediately gave Killer 12 cc of dipyrone, 10 mg of Torbugesic, and 100 mg of Rompun IV. Killer's pulse was 90 before the drugs took effect. I then passed a stomach tube, releasing just a little moderately smelly stomach gas. Next was a rectal exam that revealed a gas-distended caudal abdomen, but no impaction, displacement, or torsion was found. I then pumped a gallon of mineral oil through the stomach tube that was still in place.

The whole time Killer, whose ground manners were only marginal at best, had not moved a step. His nickname had been earned by the way he terrorized whatever horses were turned out with him. I asked Billy to walk him a bit while I decided what to do next. It was difficult to move him, but when we did get him to take a couple steps, I saw he had a worse problem than the colic. The horse barely moved because of Grade IV acute laminitis!

Killer had a throbbing digital pulse and would not allow either foot to be picked up. I gave him 15 cc of Bute IV, 8 cc of Lasix, and told Billy to point him toward a muddy area about 30 feet away where there was an overflowing water trough. I worked on his rear end with a whip, and together we managed to get him into the muddy paddock next to the trough. We tied him to the fence standing about six inches deep in soft, cool mud. I told Billy I was going home for breakfast, but I'd be back in less than an hour to recheck him before starting on the day's scheduled calls.

When I returned in about an hour, Killer had broken his leather halter and was roaming their 14-acre paddock, obviously feeling much better. I wanted to recheck his pulse, gums, and abdomen and trim his front feet, but Billy and I were unable to catch him! We tried with grain but couldn't get close enough to even get a rope around his neck. Killer felt he'd had enough medication for the day, so I told Billy I'd stop back after my day's calls and see him then.

At the end of the day, we had no more luck trying to catch him without a halter. I left Billy with instructions to please call me when he was able to get a halter on him. While the gas colic seemed resolved, I was certain he would need additional Bute and proper trimming for optimum healing of the Grade IV acute laminitis. Over the next ten days or so I drove by the farm at least a half dozen times only to see Killer roaming his muddy paddock by the road without a halter. He showed no soreness.

When the owner passed away a couple years later, a young lady purchased the green broke, now 13-year-old, gelding, to start his second career. The farrier said he showed no signs whatsoever of his severe one-day attack of acute laminitis. This case is definitely an unusual anecdote, which is dangerous to generalize from, but it is an extreme example of the benefits of allowing a horse with acute laminitis to roam free in a soft paddock. I believe the enhanced circulation to the feet from the alternating pressure of free choice, light walking is a huge advantage over the stagnant foot circulation of horses confined to a stall.

Normally, in this horse I would monitor his digital pulse daily, trim his feet properly, and expect to give the minimum effective daily dose of Bute to keep him walking comfortably and the pulse barely detectable. In thin or fit horses, the duration on this method seems to range from three to ten days. In fat, cresty, or obese horses it usually takes six to eight weeks before the endotoxins have cleared their system.

Never give more Bute than necessary for a particular case. Too much of a good thing can kill the horse. Older ponies are especially susceptible to Bute overdose ulcers, but they can also occur in young healthy horses which are given too much.

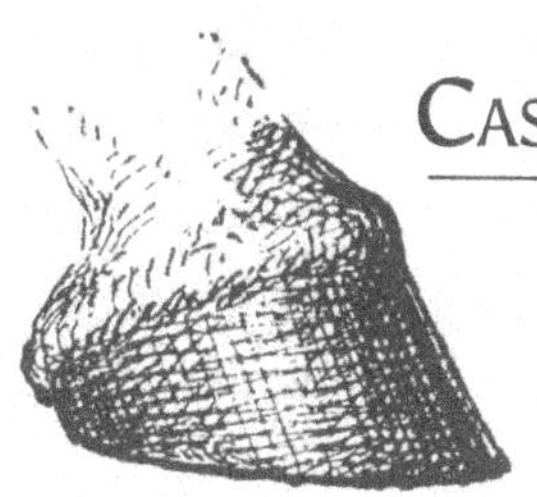

## Case Study

# "Sadie"

*Two Attacks of Very Severe Laminitis*
*3 1/2 Years Apart —*
*Both Very Quickly 100% Recovered*

I FIRST SAW SADIE ON November 9, 1991, as a Saturday afternoon emergency lameness call. She was a 6-year-old Spotted Walking Horse mare who could not move a step in her stall. She had been purchased on Tuesday as a first horse for a new family. She was shipped about 50 miles on Wednesday to her new boarding stable where the parents and daughter took turns riding her for about two hours on Thursday without any problems. They each went to work and school on Friday while Sadie stayed in her stall eating her new hay and grain. Saturday she was rocked back on her haunches in the textbook laminitis stance, the severity of which I rarely saw in my practice. She had a throbbing digital pulse in all four feet, refused to let me pick up a foot, and her back was extremely rigid and sore to touch. On top of her Grade IV acute laminitis, she also had what we called azoturia, tying up, or "Monday Morning" disease.

I immediately gave Sadie 12 cc of Bute (2.4 gm) IV and 5 cc of Lasix IV. Within a couple minutes I was able to get her to move her hindquarters over in the stall by leaning on her hips. Then I did the same thing with her shoulders, getting her to move sideways to catch her balance. Next, I gave her lead rope to Mom in the aisle while I pushed her hips and shoulders mostly sideways, but enough forward that we soon had her in the aisle. I still could not pick up a front foot, but I rasped the clinches off her front shoe nails with her feet on the ground. I was much younger and stronger in 1991, and I was next able to pick up each front foot barely long enough to pull the front shoes off. She was quickly enough improved from the drugs, movement, and shoe removal that we were able to lead her out of the barn and stand her in a large puddle in the driveway around the barn. It was about 40 degrees and had been raining all day, so she had all four feet in very cold water several inches deep.

Standing in the large puddle (even in the cold soft rain) it was easy for everyone to see her starting to relax while I continued to gather more history on the mare's first few days with her new family. Within ten minutes she stretched out and urinated what seemed like a gallon of very dark urine while standing in the puddle. While her new owners had no idea what Sadie had been eating before they bought her, both of Sadie's diseases were caused by the changes in feed earlier in the week.

Typically, laminitis shows up about 24 to 48 hours after a sudden change in feed. Sadie's laminitis most likely would have been noticed by an experienced horseman on Friday, but no responsible horse person looked at her that day. The barn help had 100 other horses to feed and clean up after on Friday. She was left in the stall all day, and every hour she stood there, the swelling, inflammation, and pain only got worse.

The tying up, "Monday Morning" disease, or azoturia is caused when a horse on heavy feed and work, such as a racehorse or workhorse gets a day off with no exercise, but with no corresponding reduction in feed intake. With working draft horses this was commonly seen when they resumed work on Monday morning. It is less common in Thoroughbreds because Thoroughbreds are usually walked on days they do not go on the track, while racing trotters and pacers are more often left in their stalls on rainy days without a reduction in their grain. In the 1970s, I was taught that it was the result of too much glycogen stored in the muscle causing the heavy muscles to release myoglobin, which is toxic to the kidneys. But the professors did not approve of the racetrack vets using Lasix for this disease. They insisted it was not caused by the kidneys, but the track vets used the diuretic to quickly reduce the excess muscle toxins in the urine and prevent renal shut-down. Later in the 1990s, researchers found some cases were genetic and created a new name—PolySaccharide Storage Myopathy, or PSSM. Lasix was frowned upon, and a very simple and easy to treat illness was turned into a mysterious and occasionally fatal disease.

Fortunately tying up was never as common as laminitis. While I saw over 1,200 cases of laminitis in 42 years, I saw less than 100 cases of tying up. Most of those were in trotters and pacers in the 1970s and '80s when there were several training farms near me. Every case of tying up I saw responded quickly to a single Lasix injection. When one of my clients left her horse with a friend while she was out of town for a week, the horse tied up and died overnight despite $600 worth of drug treatments from the friend's younger vet. When I saw everything but Lasix was given to the horse that night, I tried to discuss it with the younger vet. Even the dead horse could not cause him to question his professor or even consider why Lasix worked for so many older vets. I saw a similar case at a horse show I was working when the owners decided to take their horse to a hospital after my Lasix treatment. Another simple case was made much more complicated by several days of hospital confinement and unnecessary drugs. Sadie was the only horse I ever saw with both diseases at the same time.

After Sadie urinated in the puddle, we walked her back into the indoor arena where she walked dramatically better than when I had arrived 30 minutes earlier, and her digital pulse was far softer. I was able to hold her front feet up long enough to cut back her toes and lower her heels. She had way more hoof than she needed to walk comfortably. As we watched the daughter slowly walk her around the arena, I discussed the cause, treatment, and seriousness of laminitis with them. They knew who Secretariat was, but they didn't know he died of laminitis a few years earlier.

I left the owners with just a single 4-gram tube of Bute paste, and I asked them to give 2 grams Sunday morning and evening with as much light walking in the indoor arena as possible. With about 100 boarders, asking for free loose time in the arena was out of the question. I also inspected the hay, which was leafier than I like, so I showed them how to shake the leaves out in the aisle then give the stems back to Sadie to eat. She was to get no grain until she was off Bute and sound.

When I rechecked Sadie Monday morning, she had a very light digital pulse, came out of her stall easily, and walked out to a paddock without a problem.

I turned her loose in the paddock, and she walked very briskly without a hint of the severe soreness she had less than 48 hours earlier. Putting her back in her stall, there was no longer any detectable digital pulse. Because she was going to continue getting much more stall time than I prefer, I left the owners more of the Bute paste to be given 2 grams Monday, 1 gram Tuesday, and 1 gram Wednesday. The following week Sadie was reshod and resumed a normal feeding, riding, and stabling routine.

The farrier never saw any evidence of her brief bout with the most severe acute laminitis. This was just one more anecdote which shows you do not need to believe the researchers and professors who continue to say, "by the time a horse shows lameness from laminitis, there is already permanent damage," or that "there is no proven treatment for laminitis."

Three and a half years later Sadie had a second brief acute laminitis scare. After her first winter at the large boarding stable, Sadie moved to a more horse friendly stable, with fewer horses and more pasture. On April 29, 1995, Sadie was again found in her stall unwilling to move. This time grazing on lush spring pasture without a corresponding reduction in grain was the cause. The stable owner was a feed dealer, and he liked his boarders' horses on the plump side. Sadie was just one of several horses I had to treat for spring pasture laminitis at his stable.

Unfortunately, when I received the call that day, it was going to be 4 hours before I could get to Sadie. That was way too long to make Sadie wait for me, but there was a vet from another practice already at the barn that day. I spoke with him, and he agreed to give Sadie 10 cc of Bute and 5 cc Lasix for me. He also told me there was a farrier at the barn that morning who could remove her shoes for me. After the drugs were working and the shoes were removed Sadie's owner turned her loose in the indoor arena. They had a wash rack in the barn, so I also asked them to hose her front feet for ten minutes every hour until I got there.

When I arrived later that afternoon, Sadie was wandering around the arena on her own, showing no lameness at all. I could still feel a mild digital pulse. I squared her toes to ease her breakover in the sand and lowered her heels a little with my rasp. Like 3 1/2 years earlier, I left just one 4-gram tube of Bute to be given in progressively lower doses that week. She was reshod and back on the trails the next week, having survived a second bout of Grade IV acute laminitis with zero permanent damage. It is NOT a complicated disease!

# ~SECTION V~

## Delayed, Second Opinion Cases

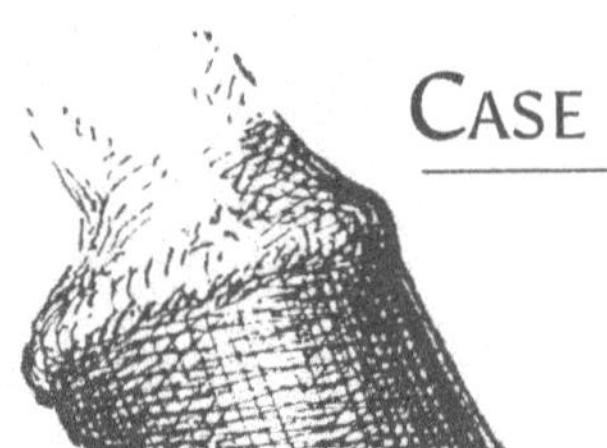

# Case Study

## "Fame"

### *Back from the brink*

This case was previously published in *EQUUS* magazine (34)

"FAME" IS RETOLD BRIEFLY HERE, not so much for its teaching value, but because it was, like Stepper (pages 68-72) and Sandy McDaniel (pages 116-121), one of the most dramatic examples where I was called far too late, well after rotation and permanent damage was underway, yet the horse was restored to drug free soundness with very simple treatment. Founder is never as easy to cure as it is to prevent, as it was for Splash and Buster. Like too many others, Fame was misdiagnosed during the acute stage of his laminitis by a very experienced veterinarian.

I received a very unusual call for an "emergency second opinion" on January 16, 1999, an extremely cold Saturday morning in Chicago. It was from Mickey, an excellent client whose sister's horse had been going straight downhill after a week of treatment, despite being seen twice by her veterinarian. Now they could not even get him out of his stall at the boarding stable. The 30-year, well-respected equine practitioner had told her on his second visit that he did not know what the problem was, but "it looked like" her 23-year-old retired American Saddlebred show horse, now trail riding buddy, "may have suffered a stroke!" Refusing to come out of his stall on Saturday morning sounded over the phone to me like acute laminitis, so I told her I could be at the barn in 30 minutes.

I had never seen Fame before, but he was obviously in severe distress in his undersized box stall (8'x10'). He was very wobbly as we forced him out into the adjacent indoor arena. He acted very much like his feet were killing him, but where I expected to feel a throbbing digital pulse, none was detectable.

Listening to his heart I could barely hear it beating weakly. His gums were pale with a very poor capillary refill. He had a blank look as he would alternately lift a rear foot off the ground and stand on three legs. He refused to let me pick up either front foot.

I believe Fame already had the most severe Grade IV acute laminitis in all four feet with likely active rotation and/or sinking underway after at least a week in his stall. He was shod all around with rather long feet, reminiscent of his show horse days. I gave him Bute IV right away and fortunately there was a horseshoer at the barn who helped remove his shoes. If a horse could say thank you with his body language, Fame did it when his shoes were finally off. We walked him a little in the very soft rubberized arena and everyone could see the horse relaxing, if not actually smiling.

After a few more minutes of light walking, I was able to hold a front foot up long enough to get about 1⁄2 inch off the front of his $4^+$-inch toes. This eased his break-over considerably. I also took about 1⁄2 inch off his heels to get his frog a little closer to the soft rubberized arena. I had a long conversation with his owner, who lived and worked in the city five days a week, and the barn owners who would be responsible for him during the week. I agreed to check him myself twice a week, as needed. Mickey said after I left that Saturday morning that Fame laid down flat at one end of the arena looking like he was dead while the other horses worked quietly at the other end of the arena. Her sisters told her that was the first relief he had had all week from the intense foot pain.

When I rechecked Fame Monday, his heart sounded much better, and he had a significant, but not throbbing digital pulse. The much better heartbeat told me Fame had actually been in shock from the pain two days earlier.

Fame's recovery went as expected with the minimum effective daily dose of Bute. I trimmed back his toes and heels a little more each week until we had a normal trail horse foot rather than a long-gaited horse foot. I believe he received a total of 99 grams of Bute over the next eight weeks of tapering Bute doses. He had only one brief setback where he was worse than on my previous visit. I found out that they had run out of his grass hay and gone back to alfalfa for him that week. My new instructions were to give him no alfalfa until he was walking sound and off Bute. When he was down to 1 gram of Bute per day, we would occasionally clap our hands while he was loose in the arena, and it was thrilling to watch him throw his tail over his back and hit his show gait.

Fame was back on the trails that summer, but three years later, after he had moved to a different stable even farther from my normal practice radius, Fame suffered a relapse of his laminitis in August 2002. Again, it started out mild, and a different, but also very experienced 30-year equine practitioner attributed his mild soreness to "normal arthritis" in the then 26-year-old Fame. A week later Fame's horseshoer told Mickey he thought it might be laminitis. I made the hour drive through heavy suburban traffic the next day and confirmed it absolutely was laminitis. It was far milder than three years earlier, but if ignored would have gotten worse. As it was, it took almost three weeks before he was back to normal. His recovery took longer than necessary because of a most uncooperative stable owner who absolutely forbid any horses being turned loose in her arena. Fame again had a very undersized box stall, and a very small turnout paddock. Mickey did have a dump truck bring in a load of sand for his turnout paddock, but he was only in it about eight hours a day, versus sixteen hours a day in the tiny stall.

The saddest end of all was that ten days after recovering from the laminitis Fame died of colic. On my last visit to pronounce his laminitis over, I gave Fame a "conditionally approved" West Nile vaccine in the face of a huge epidemic that fall. I had 12 horses with West Nile Virus (WNV) in September and October 2002, and three of them died. Most of them needed help getting up several times a day as we struggled to keep them comfortable and steady while they fought the virus.

However, four of the first 50 horses I vaccinated for WNV died of colic within ten days of being vaccinated. Fame was one of those four. He went to a clinic for the unresponsive colic, and while they drained gallons of reflux from his stomach several times a day, he did not recover. His laminitis did not return with the colic. I absolutely believe the first version of that vaccine was much harsher than necessary.

Why did two very experienced equine practitioners miss Fame's early signs of laminitis? It happens far more often than anyone wants to admit. How many of us got 100% on all our tests in school? Certainly not me! The difference is that after graduation there is no teacher to point out your errors. Not all laminitis cases have the same classic signs. You have to suspect it before you can look for it, and then you might have to use several different diagnostic tests or observations before you can make the diagnosis. X-rays can only show if coffin bone movement has started. Far too often acute laminitis is missed precisely because there has not yet been movement. That is when a careful physical exam must make the diagnosis to prevent founder!

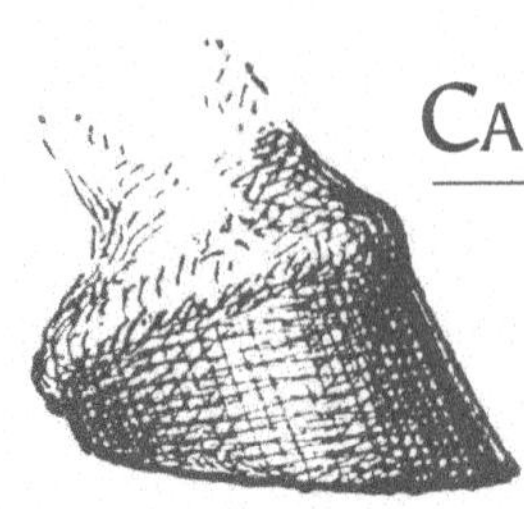

# Case Study

## "Tango"

*Fatal 25-Year-Old American Saddlebred Gelding*

TANGO WAS ADOPTED AT AGE 23 from the Humane Society which had rescued him in 1990. The new owner was a 72-year-old man who had been very active with his daughter's six to eight Appaloosa show horses for about ten years until her college graduation. Then the daughter got a job, moved away from home, and most of her horses were sold. Dad still had the barn and arena in his backyard, but the two remaining horses were not enough activity for him, so he adopted the retired Saddlebred no one else wanted.

Bob always called me very promptly for any problem with his horses. He was an excellent client, very intelligent, never tight with money, and he made up for his marginal horsemanship by being a very good listener. He easily understood anything I explained to him, but none of his daughter's horses had ever suffered a single bout of laminitis, so Bob never had the occasion to discuss how I diagnosed and treated the disease.

Bob noticed Tango was a little lame one Saturday morning. He suspected it might be an early hoof abscess, which he had seen several times in other horses. The farrier was scheduled to trim the horses that day, so Bob decided to let him have a look at Tango rather than call me. Tom, one of my favorite farriers for over 30 years, recognized it was mild laminitis rather than an abscess.

Tom decided to try the latest advice from Kentucky at that time. He nailed three 6-degree wedge pads on Tango's front feet. This raised his angle 18 degrees "to relieve the pull of the tendon on the back of the coffin bone." This seemed to Bob and Tom to provide some relief. Tango was in his stall every night but walked around the paddocks every day in his new platform shoes.

Two weeks later I was called for standard spring booster vaccinations. I was shocked to see the elevated shoes on the old, retired horse, and offended by Bob's explanation that this was the latest treatment for laminitis. I had provided 24/7 veterinary care for his horses' cuts, colics, foaling, etc., for over ten years, but I was not even called for my favorite disease. Tango seemed to be getting around okay, so while I did not agree with the built-up shoes, I did not insist they should be removed immediately.

A couple weeks later Tango was progressively more sore and I was called back. I then removed the shoes, stopped the alfalfa, upped the Bute, and asked for 24-hour turnout in the indoor arena. Since the daughter had left home a few years earlier, a variety of vehicles and farm equipment were now stored in the arena. Bob would turn Tango loose during the day, but each night he had to be put back in his stall. Within a week I was asked to put Tango to sleep. It was simply too much work for a 72-year-old man who still worked at his engineering office every day.

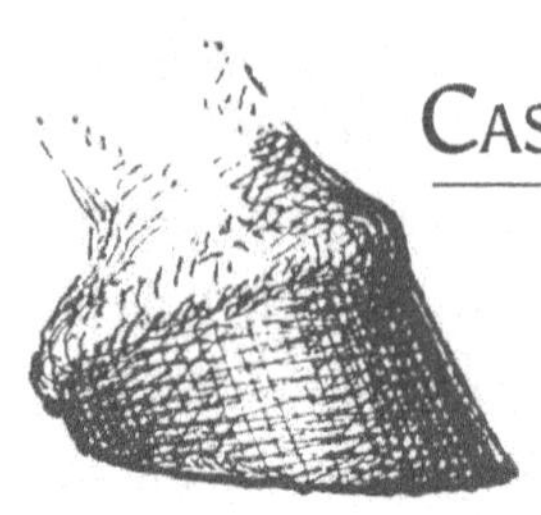

## Case Study

# "Sandy McDaniel"

### *550 Grams of Bute Over 25 Weeks to Save a Life*

SANDY MCDANIEL WAS A 22-YEAR-OLD Paint mare, who may have been 250 pounds overweight, when I first saw her as a third opinion laminitis case on June 18, 2001. She had Grade IV laminitis symptoms for ten days and was being treated with banamine, acepromazine, pergolide, nitroglycerine, stall confinement, egg bar shoes and silicone pads at a local hospital. She had also been on 30 isoxsuprine tablets and aspirin daily the past six years for navicular disease diagnosed in 1995. Furthermore, she received 10cc regumate daily for suspected cystic ovaries, which reportedly caused four mild colics in the spring of 2000. I considered her heavily medicated when I first saw her.

The first vet had examined her for lameness four weeks earlier on May 23. With an ultrasound, her lameness was diagnosed as a strained suspensory ligament. This was suspect because all the mare had been doing was grazing her lush pasture nonstop. The first vet prescribed 1 gram Bute daily, 2 weeks stall confinement with daily hand walking (at least she was taken off the excellent pasture), a DMSO sweat on the ligament, and extended egg bar shoes for her front feet. All this was done faithfully by Sandy's owner, Pam, for two weeks until she called for a recheck because the mare was only getting worse.

On June 8th, with Sandy refusing to walk and reportedly leaning back on her haunches, the attending vet diagnosed laminitis, and treated her with more Bute, Banamine, Acepromazine, and DMSO sweats. Because his portable X-ray machine was not working, he asked Pam to bring her into their vet clinic ten miles away the next day for radiographs. The vets at the clinic could see that the coffin bone had already started to rotate and drop on June 9th. They admitted her to their hospital.

After three more days of stall confinement and the various medications listed above, Sandy was X-rayed again, on June 12th. I stopped to see both sets of radiographs before my second visit to Sandy. Her coffin bone clearly moved during her first three days of stall confinement at the clinic. On her 5th day at the hospital, June 14th, Sandy was taken out of her stall, directly into the indoor arena at the clinic. She went down in the sand and refused to get up for two hours. Her prognosis was so poor that they discussed euthanasia while she lay there. The egg bar shoes were finally pulled her sixth day at the clinic and the next day Pam took Sandy home "barely able to walk." She had silicone pads on her front feet and Styrofoam pads on the rear feet. Over the weekend it was obvious to Pam that Sandy was more comfortable in her sand paddock, or on her lush clover pasture than she was in her stall. Incredibly, no one had yet explained the connection between obesity, lush pasture, and laminitis to this first-time horse owner!

I was called for the first time on Monday, June 18. This was ten days after the laminitis was obvious to everyone, and 28 days after lameness had started, and she was taken off her lush pasture for stall rest and hand walking (but continued on grain) for the suspected "suspensory problem." Despite her daily battery of medications, Sandy had Grade IV laminitis. She had strong digital pulse pressure in all four feet, and she was barely able to stand on three feet for a few seconds at a time while I squared off her toes in front to ease breakover and take some of the strain off the toe laminae. I left the taped-on pads in front, prescribed 2 grams of Bute twice a day, stopped the banamine, flunixin (another anti-inflammatory), acepromazine, nitroglycerin (both vasodilators), Cushing's medication, all grain, alfalfa hay, and especially her lush spring clover pasture. I also asked for 24-hour open access to the sand paddock and her deeply bedded box stall—at Sandy's choice. Having only one other horse in the barn made this workable. Unlike some Paints and Quarter Horses, Sandy was blessed with large, round hooves which were in good proportion to her very large body size.

Before my next visit I stopped by the previous vet's clinic to check the X-rays taken June 9 and 12. They were not marked or measured, but there appeared to be 3° or 4° rotation in each front foot a week earlier, and she was obviously not yet stabilized.

Upon rechecking Sandy on June 21, I found her lying in the sand working her way through an enormous pile of grass hay. When she reluctantly got up, there was no improvement in her pain level. I gave her 2 grams of Bute IV in addition to the 2 grams orally she was receiving twice a day. This was more than I would normally consider safe, but her size and pain level made taking the risk of overdose ulcers necessary. I also inspected the cherry tree about 15 feet outside her sand paddock. Sure enough, the overhanging leaves and branches had been eaten as high and far over the fence as Sandy's neck could reach. I had assumed that Sandy's laminitis was due to obesity, grain, and extremely good spring clover pastures, however, when they were removed, she apparently started grazing the cherry tree, which may have been even worse.

It was still extremely difficult to get Sandy to hold up a front foot for more than 20 seconds at a time. By alternating front feet, we managed to replace her silicone sole pads with the diapers and duct tape over iodine and Epsom salts, which I used to optimize moisture (too moist and soft can be even worse than too dry and hard). The iodine also discourages infectious abscesses while the hoof is suffering from inadequate circulation. Due to her size and poor pain relief, I increased her daily Bute to 5 gm in divided doses.

My third visit was three days later on Sunday, June 24. She was still Grade IV, but we eventually managed to get the diapers changed. I rasped her heels down a bit and was pleased to find she still had firm soles, and there was no gross evidence yet of sinking coffin bones. I usually prescribe unlimited grass hay, but Sandy had such a good appetite, and she did not appear to have lost a pound yet. We had to put her on a diet, so we were forced to limit her to two flakes of hay three times a day.

The next day she was still not responding quickly enough, so I raised the Bute to 3 grams twice a day and had Pam put one flake of hay in each corner of her sand paddock to encourage her to walk more in the sand, which would stimulate better circulation in her feet. There was a large pile of sand in one corner, but it was thin and hard in other areas, so I asked Pam if she could get some help to spread it around to a more uniform depth of about 4 inches all around the paddock. She and her good friend, Barb, who often helped change the diapers, moved sand with a wheelbarrow all weekend. Since moist sand seemed softer than dry sand, they also put the sprinkler on the sand paddock.

X-rays on June 25 amazingly showed her coffin bones had not moved significantly since June 12, despite two weeks of severe pain and very poor circulation to her laminae. Walking in the paddock seemed to be doing more good than the stall confinement at the hospital.

While Pam and Barb worked with Sandy's feet daily, my next visit wasn't until July 2, when Pam was out of town. Unbelievably, Pam's border had turned Sandy out on her clover laden pasture that morning! I found her walking significantly better, and able to stand on three feet much easier for the diaper changes, but I gave her a gallon of mineral oil via stomach tube hoping to prevent the day's clover gorging from causing another relapse.

The oil purging worked, as we had no setback. The Bute was dropped to 5 grams for the next ten days, then 4 grams as she continued to improve. She was walking much better in the deep sand, and picking up her feet more easily for trimming, but it still hurt her to turn around in the barn aisle on the rubber mats.

Pivoting puts torque on the laminae, which will be obviously painful even with mild laminitis. As the hoof grows during treatment, I normally trim the front feet more frequently, rasping back the toe, and keeping the heels low to keep the slightly rotated coffin bone level with the ground. I also try very hard to keep enough wall at the quarters to prevent ground pressure on the middle of the sole. There is important circulation between the coffin bone and soul which can easily be compressed if the sole is too close to the ground, or packed with dry, hard mud, or ice and snow in the winter. The diapers and duct tape prevent the packing and encourage walking.

By the time I visited Sandy on July 12 she was comfortable enough to drop the Bute to 4 grams per day, however after trimming her as described above she got worse instead of better, and we had to go back up to 5 grams per day. The rest of July she received between 4 and 6 grams of Bute daily, depending on the degree of soreness. By July 31 she had slowly lost about 50 pounds, but she was back up to 6 grams of Bute, so we X-rayed her again. The X-rays still showed no further rotation, but possibly a little sinking of the coffin bone within the hoof capsule.

On August 2, I was able to open a clear, serious abscess at the toe of her right front hoof. I consider this a non-infectious abscess due to pressure necrosis of the sensitive tissues under the coffin bone.

We treated Sandy's abscess with the iodine and Epsom salts under the diaper and duct tape. On August 6, the left front hoof was starting to show a similar suspicious soft spot at the toe. And on August 9, we opened that and got a thin, bloody drainage. We had to go up to 6 grams of Bute for one day, then 5 grams for three days, before leveling off at 4 grams per day from August 10 through September 28. I checked on her only twice in that time, noting on August 23 that she appeared to be down about 100 pounds since the start of her laminitis, and that for the first time I was able to feel one of her ribs—still a long way from actually seeing a rib! On 2 grams of Bute morning and evening she was walking quite well in her sand paddock.

Sandy had another bout with pressure under the left front toe in mid-September, which was treated with icthammol ointment under the diaper, without having to go above 4 grams of Bute per day. On September 29 she was dropped to 3 grams of Bute, and on October 1 she was doing well enough to drop the Bute to 2 grams per day. I did not see Sandy again until October 30. Pam had faithfully kept a daily calendar of her progress, medication, and only two brief setbacks. When I saw her on October 30 it was the first time I had seen good enough soles under her feet in over four months to leave her feet unwrapped! She was moving, turning, and changing directions rather quickly, so I advised dropping to just 1 gm Bute per day.

On November 13, after 25 weeks of daily Bute (a total of 550 grams in 167 days) the Bute was stopped for good. Sandy was now a svelte 1,200 pounds, her girth was shortened five holes, and she could run and play in her pasture again. Pam had her pasture sprayed twice that summer to kill the clover.

The following spring and summer Sandy was limited to two hours per day on pasture—and those two hours her mouth rarely left the ground. She was a world champion eating machine. Nevertheless, she never had another bout of laminitis and had no more Bute into her 30s!

Sandy's treatment took about three to four times longer than the typical six- to eight-week laminitis recovery I see with similar fat or cresty horses. This was probably due to a combination of factors such as 1) the delay in recognizing the laminitis until she was rocked back and immobile, 2) the further delay in receiving appropriate treatment after the week at the clinic with stall rest, vasodilators, and egg bar shoes, 3) the triple whammy of the cherry tree, after clover and grain obesity, and 4) the repeated abscess complications.

Without the outstanding nursing, the free choice sand paddock, the minimum effective daily dose of Bute (in this extreme case up to 6 grams on really bad days), the daily diapering of her feet, and the strict diet, there is little doubt she would have been humanely euthanized.

The very high Bute dosage (101 consecutive days between 4 and 6 grams daily) would seem dangerously excessive to most veterinarians. In Sandy's case, I felt it was absolutely necessary to control the inflammation and swelling in her feet, to allow room for as much fresh blood as possible to save her severely stressed laminae.

# ~SECTION VI~

## Complicated Cases with Severe Causes

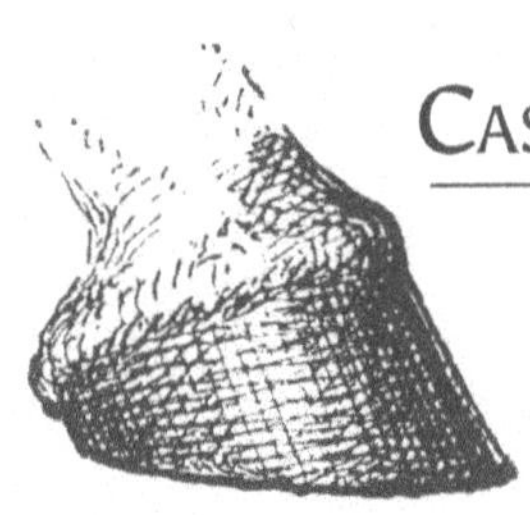

## Case Study

# "Polly"

### *Retained Placenta, New Foal a Year Later*

I WAS CALLED TO LOOK at Polly, an 8-year-old Belgian brood mare because of sudden lameness. Her owner, Bill, had been taking care of horses for about 60 years, and he felt she might have a hoof abscess.

I could see by walking Polly that she was sore on both front feet. She also had a 3-to-4-day old foal beside her. Polly had increased digital pulse pressure in both front feet, and she was sensitive to tapping on her front hoof walls with the hoof testers. She never liked to have her feet picked up, so I didn't try very hard to pick them up for the hoof testers. She definitely had acute laminitis.

I asked Bill if she had passed her afterbirth right away. He said, "Oh sure, it was gone when I got here that morning." She had foaled out in the pasture several nights earlier. I took Polly's temperature, and it was 103.8° F. She had no vaginal discharge, but I put on a long sleeve and went through her cervix. Sure enough I brought out a 3 or 4 day old placenta covered with pus.

Bill felt terrible as I inserted some sulfaurea antibiotic boluses into her uterus. I also gave her 35 cc of penicillin and 12 cc of Bute because she weighed close to 2,000 pounds. I then told Bill that mild exercise would be good, for both her feet and her uterus.

When I stopped to check Polly the next day, there was no sign of the laminitis, and her temperature was 100.5° F. Bill had slept in his pickup truck the night before, getting up to ride the mare once around the pond every hour! I gave her another 20 cc of Penicillin and 12 cc of Bute.

On the third day she was quite normal, and I simply inserted a couple more sulfa-urea antibiotic boluses into her uterus. Believe it or not, in a couple months she was back in foal, with no lingering effects of the laminitis whatsoever.

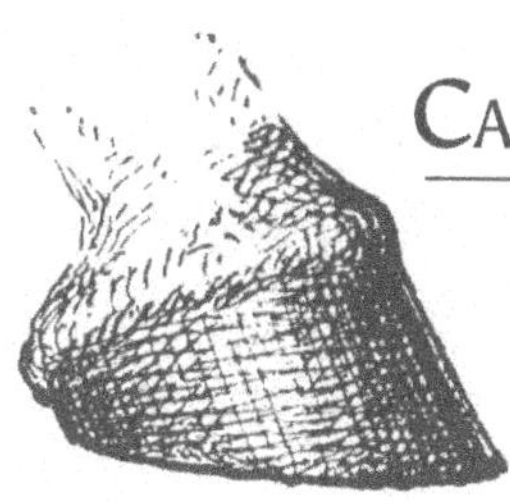

# Case Study

## "Linda"

### *Severe Dystocia, 75 Hour Retained Placenta, and Fatal Peritonitis*

LINDA'S STORY IS VERY SAD, but it must be told, and included with my other severe laminitis stories, such as Joey, Sandy McDaniel, Fame, Caesar, Sunny, Dixie, Polly, Sadie, Killer, etc. (all real names of really very bad acute laminitis cases). With the others, this case report starkly illustrates the point that no matter how severe the triggering cause of laminitis, the ongoing illness, the Obel grade of laminitis itself, or the size of the horse; the basic treatment principle of restoring and maintaining optimum circulation ASAP (while eliminating the triggering cause) still works. Of course, it works much quicker if the cause can be eliminated and if correct treatment starts before the compressed and oxygen starved laminae have allowed the coffin bone to start moving within the hoof.

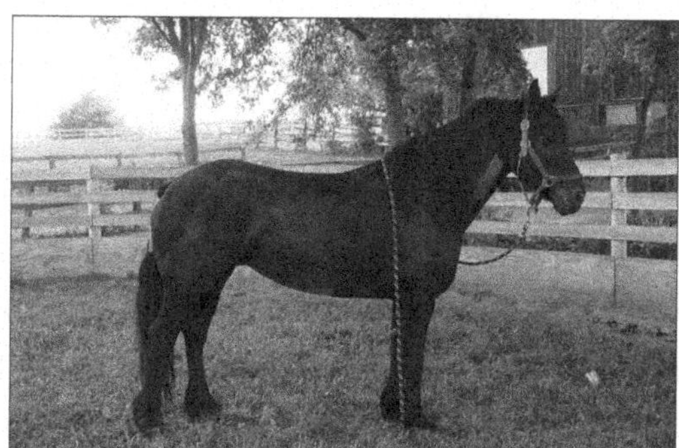

*Linda*

The names and a few minor identifying details in this particular story have been changed to protect the owner's privacy, and because the other veterinarians involved with Linda's case still do not share my belief that laminitis is basically a very simple disease to treat regardless of the underlying cause. The hard facts which affected the course of this case, and which do not compromise the owner's or the veterinarians' identities, have not been changed at all.

I have never practiced in a hospital, however over 42 years, I did, on a regular basis, refer well over 400 difficult cases with seriously ill or injured horses (only two with laminitis) to four different university hospitals and seven different private equine hospitals within reasonable driving distance of my practice area. The driving distance for my clients' horses was often the deciding factor in emergencies, however the specific expertise and relationships with the various clinicians available over the 42 years also determined which clinic was chosen for a specific case.

It is because horses with laminitis have such a high complication and fatality rate in most university hospitals that the general public is told laminitis is such a mysterious and deadly disease. The university vets, who submit most of the articles and sit on the peer review panels and editorial boards, often control what the veterinary journals will publish. Private practitioners' reports are usually dismissed as insignificant anecdotes. A two-year university trial with 20 ponies is considered scientific evidence, but over 42 years treating over 1,200 horses and ponies with laminitis (some individual horses for more than 30 years each) is not considered "evidence-based medicine." Field vets' decisions are based on the evidence we are presented with every day in the field.

Some reports (28) have shown that approximately 50% of horses with laminitis in hospitals die or are euthanized, while the largest farm survey (30) shows only a little over 5% of horses with laminitis die or are euthanized on farms. Two published reports, one experimental (35) and one clinical (36) have shown 100% recovery for horses treated properly before the damage has started. My personal rate is barely over 2% choosing euthanasia because of laminitis. In every one of my laminitis deaths either I, the owners, or another involved party "dropped the ball." Two published reviews of 40 cases of naturally occurring laminitis in Pennsylvania (29) and 60 cases at a large practice in England (37) both showed 25% deaths due to laminitis over the approximately four years the horses were followed. This leads me to believe that while the seriousness and severity of the underlying disease may be crucial factors in most diseases, the treatment theory and facility chosen have a larger impact on laminitis survival rates. I have never believed the excuses that some horses with laminitis are doomed regardless of the treatment chosen.

Many veterinarians in hospitals maintain that the different laminitis survival rates are because horses in hospitals "are so much sicker" than the general population on the farm. Most university clinicians refuse to discuss these different fatality rates. While Dr. Bill Moyer would discuss it with me, in the end he chose to "agree to disagree." I usually learn much more from the horses that die than from the survivors. Writing about the details of deaths such as Linda are especially difficult for most vets, but so necessary if we want to learn from our mistakes.

Linda was a very stout 5-year-old purebred European sport horse mare. While she was short for her breed at 15.2 hands, she was heavily muscled, long-bodied, and thick-boned, and weighed close to 1,400 pounds. She was purchased by my client as an unbroken, but in-foal, 3-year-old. She had her first purebred foal at 4, was rebred and then green-broke after she weaned her first colt.

My client Carol, arriving home after a late Monday night meeting, checked on Linda just after midnight two weeks before she was due to have her second foal. Carol found Linda in distress and immediately called me saying she wasn't sure if the mare had a bad colic or was in labor, but she was violent and needed me right away. After I dressed and was on my way to her home 20 miles away, I called Carol back on my cell phone. The mare was indeed in labor and had the foal's head out, but she was too violent getting up and down for the owner to safely offer any assistance, or even control the mare. I arrived about 12:40 am and the mare was down halfway out the doorway into the paddock connected to her stall. The foal's head showed no sign of life, and the gums were dark blue. Carol said that when the foal's head first appeared about 30 minutes earlier, it did blink and appeared alive, but after the mare had gotten up and down several times and bumped the foal on the walls, she was also sure it was dead. No feet or legs were in sight. I tried to enter the mare's vagina in search of the legs, but this caused Linda to immediately jump up and pace in and out of the stall before crashing again. About this time the farrier, who also had been called for emergency help, arrived to offer some assistance in controlling the mare.

The third time Linda got up after crashing, I tranquilized her with Rompun and Torbugesic, and the farrier was able to control her while I again searched for the foal's legs as she stood and strained. This was a powerful and very deep bodied mare who strongly resisted me and pushed back very hard against my efforts to repel the foal and locate a leg. I knew right away that I was overmatched in the barn and that the mare's best chance was at a hospital where general anesthesia, a C-section, or even an embryotomy would be safer options. We had the mare loaded on a trailer within five more minutes. The owner wanted me to ride with her to the hospital, but instead I agreed to follow her trailer to the hospital. On the way I called ahead and spoke with an intern who lived at the hospital. I gave her an estimated 1:45 am arrival time. I told her that the mare was extremely difficult, and that she would very possibly need either a C-section or an embryotomy to deliver the dead foal. I asked if she would please try to have the surgeon at the hospital when we arrived, rather than their standard practice of waiting until they had evaluated the patient before calling in the surgeon.

I was very pleased to see the surgeon drive through the hospital gate immediately before us at 1:50 am. The two interns were set up and well prepared for every possibility I had described, including anesthesia, sterile surgery packs, OB chains, and a Gigly wire for a possible embryotomy. Linda was unloaded directly into the padded pre-op stall where the surgeon searched for the foal's legs for less than a minute, before meeting powerful resistance and deciding to put the mare on the surgical table under general anesthesia. While the tranquilizer and trailer ride had stopped the violent labor, she still pushed powerfully against human efforts to reposition the foal. Linda went down smoothly, was intubated, and hoisted by straps and an electric winch attached to an I-beam which allowed her to be placed on the surgical table with V-shaped supports holding her directly upside down. The table was then hydraulically tilted to allow gravity to help repel the foal back into the mare while the surgeon tried to locate and expose the front legs for delivery. This was an incredibly difficult and slow process which took about an hour to expose just one front leg.

Throughout the process, the two resident vets managed the anesthesia at the head, a very experienced and capable technician assisted the surgeon at the rear end, and a visiting vet student was available to retrieve any supplies or equipment needed by anyone. I was mostly left to observe, ask questions, make suggestions, relay progress and options to the owner who waited in an adjacent room, and occasionally hold a leg out of the way. As the surgeon passed an hour of extremely difficult pushing and straining to retrieve and expose the legs, I offered several times to give him some relief and see if I might have any better luck at retrieving the second leg. I am no expert, but I have had to perform such manipulations on awake mares in barns probably a dozen times or more. I was well aware of how difficult and exhausting the work could be, and I knew this was an especially difficult case.

The surgeon remarked several times that he felt the foal's legs were severely contracted which was making it so difficult to extend them and pull the foal's feet out for a normal delivery. Since no one believed the foal had been alive since we arrived, I several times suggested cutting the foal's head and neck off with the embryotomy wire that was in the surgical room if he chose to use it. I thought this would allow more room for the surgeon to go in after the legs. This idea was vetoed because the surgeon felt jagged neck bones could do more harm to the already bruised vaginal walls. The suggestion to cut the other front leg off was originally vetoed for the same reason. Sometime after an hour of general anesthesia the mare's abdomen was shaved and prepped for a possible Caesarian while the surgeon continued his determined struggle to expose the second front leg. As we approached two hours of general anesthesia, the embryotomy wire was finally used to amputate the second leg through the contracted knee joint. The technician and I then pulled the foal out with chains he had placed on both the long and the short leg. The dead foal was out within a few minutes of amputating the leg. The foal's legs were indeed severely contracted, not just at the fetlocks and knees, but the elbows, and shoulders were also severely contracted and could not be extended. If the foal had been born alive, even by a timely C-section, I doubt very much if it ever would have been able to stand.

I left shortly after 4:00 am, before the mare was taken to recovery. The surgeon stayed at the hospital through the difficult recovery from anesthesia, then worked a normal day with two hours' sleep (I got one more hour in bed before the phone started ringing again). I received periodic reports from the owner the next two days that Linda was up and about, eating, running a moderate fever, but had still not passed her placenta. I called the hospital and spoke to the surgeon about the retained placenta. He assured me they were flushing her uterus with an antibiotic solution daily, administering oxytocin several times a day (a total of eight injections increasing up to 5 cc at a time over three days), treating her vaginal wounds topically after each flush, monitoring her vital signs throughout the day and night, and keeping her on broad spectrum systemic antibiotics and Banamine. He felt the retained placenta was due to a hormone imbalance associated with pre-term delivery. A CBC taken on day three, at 53 hours after delivery, showed a WBC of just 2,000, including 580 neutrophils and 200 band cells. Her circulating white cells had been overwhelmed with bacterial infection.

The mare finally released the putrid placenta on day four, about 75 hours after delivery. The hospital chart shows the intern repeatedly checked and found no increased digital pulse pressure the three prior days of the retained placenta. The morning the placenta was passed, 10 mg of Acepromazine was given orally and continued BID throughout her hospital stay. While the intern noted the mare had "difficulty getting up" later that morning after she had passed the placenta, and she "seemed stressed outside" that afternoon, the intern first noticed the increased digital pulse and laminitis lameness 24 hours later. That was early Saturday morning when the owner called me again to report Linda's laminitis. Carol had previously had two minor bouts of laminitis in one of her older geldings which we had quickly resolved both times. She knew I treated laminitis differently from most vets, and she asked me to drive to the clinic Saturday morning to check her mare and be sure they were treating her laminitis appropriately.

The surgeon was in the middle of a colic surgery when I arrived about 8:00 am Saturday. Three other vets were busy with other cases in the hospital, so I said hello and went to Linda's stall by myself. She was standing, eating hay under her feed tub at the front of the stall. Like in all the other stalls, the barn man had swept the shavings back from the front 1/3 of the stall to make it easier for the horses to eat dropped feed with less waste, and to keep the hospital aisle cleaner. Unfortunately, the hospital's neatness protocol did not help cushion Linda's feet on the hard floors. She had an easily detectable digital pulse at all four fetlocks. She would not allow either front foot to be picked up, and when forced to move to the back of the stall, she was obviously sore in all four feet. Her laminitis was Obel Grade IV, as she would not walk without being forced. I pushed her to the back of the stall, kicked some of the shavings toward the front, and waited.

The intern assigned to Linda did come back to check on her, offered her observations on the case since the embryotomy four days earlier, and pretty much politely ignored my thoughts on treating acute laminitis. The hospital had just one grass/dirt/mud (depending on rain) round pen for any horse which needed to be turned out. Linda had been getting a turn outside most days with the retained placenta, and they planned to continue that with the laminitis. This was better than most hospitals which keep horses confined to their stall once laminitis starts.

The intern gave me Linda's seven-page medical chart to review while I was waiting for the surgeon to discuss her laminitis treatment. The surgeon finished his surgery about 9:30, then came back to flush Linda's uterus and treat the vaginal wounds with an antibiotic and steroid cream.

We discussed his plan for her acute laminitis treatment. I preferred 24-hour turnout with frequent cold hosing. He agreed to daily turnout of unspecified time with hosing on the way to and from the single round pen. I believe Acepromazine, as a vasodilator, interferes with the horse's intrinsic attempt to restore as much circulation to the swollen laminae as possible. He believed 10 mg of Acepromazine orally twice a day was sufficient to soften the digital pulse pressure. He said if she stayed at his hospital, that's what she would get—if we didn't want her to get it we'd have to take her home. I believe in the minimum effective daily dose of Bute, which in a mare this size could be as high as 6 grams some days. He believed alternating 2 grams of Bute with 10 cc of Banamine was safer and sufficient. I believe acute laminitis, regardless of the cause, is really a very simple disease to treat if you can eliminate the cause (presumably the 75-hour retained placenta here). He told me that was "ignorant," and there was nothing simple or predictable about laminitis.

After Linda's treatment and our discussion in the stall, the surgeon slowly led her to the round pen while I followed and encouraged her from behind. She left the stall extremely reluctant and sore, but she got a little better the farther we walked. We stopped at the end of the hospital to cold hose her feet for a few minutes, and she walked even better when we got to the round pen. The walking absolutely improved the circulation to her feet, and the cold hosing probably reduced the inflammation and numbed the feet somewhat.

After I left, the surgeon and I both called Carol separately to give her progress reports and our different opinions on the best treatment of her severe laminitis. The treatment of the uterine infection and damaged vagina was not in question. I am a totally unqualified surgeon, and I'm only confident with very basic internal medicine. But I've felt my entire career that acute laminitis is the simplest and most predictable disease I get to treat. I was convinced that with the treatment plan proposed at the hospital, Linda was headed for disaster. I believed she needed to be outside and moving 24/7 to maintain the circulation critical to her laminae. Even an hour in a stall will raise the digital pulse pressure in a horse with acute laminitis, indicating insufficient oxygen to the laminae. Acepromazine does not improve circulation to the inflamed laminae, it dilates the constricted pastern and fetlock arterioles, defeating the horse's sympathetic attempt to overcome the oxygen deficit and the increased pressure of laminar inflammation.

I do not normally take patients on our small farm, as I do not have any hospital facilities, and I do not have paid employees to watch my farm or patients while I'm off visiting other clients' farms. Nevertheless, I strongly believed Linda would have a much better chance to win her battle with acute laminitis in our sand round pen 24/7, with whatever dose of Bute was necessary, and without Acepromazine; then she would have in and out of a hospital stall, with limited Bute, and with Ace twice a day. I urged Carol to bring Linda to our farm. She decided to keep Linda at the hospital for another day.

Linda was even more sore Sunday morning, with a "bounding digital pulse" and having trouble moving at all in the stall "without falling down," so Carol called to ask if she could now bring her to our farm. She arrived at 11:00 am Sunday, and I was unable to pick up either front foot to check her soles when she got off the trailer. By the time we had gotten her to the round pen, she was walking better, and I was able to remove the hard packed mud from the day before at the hospital's round pen. I started her on 6 cc Lasix for laminar edema and 2 more grams Bute paste for inflammation and pain, while Carol cold hosed her feet in the round pen. We brought my wife's 32-year-old gelding into the round pen with her to stimulate her to move around more and help eat the grass which had grown in the 10-inch bed of sand. My younger son had also spent considerable time Saturday when we had expected to receive Linda, shoveling the sand off the outside wall to make the outer walking track softer and deeper.

We periodically repeated the hosing throughout the day. Linda lost interest in following the older gelding around the round pen, so we brought in a younger and feistier mare to stimulate her to move more. After a few initial snorts they also pretty much ignored each other. I gave Linda 2 more grams of Bute IV at 8:30 pm as she was still "very sore." That was a total of 6 grams for that day, including the 2 grams she had received at the hospital that morning. We had switched her antibiotic to 12 tabs (960 mg) sulfamethoxazole-trimethoprim (SMZ-TMP) orally BID.

At 5:30 am Monday (dawn in June), Linda was lying comfortably in the sand on her chest with her head up and alert. Surprisingly, she let me hose her feet while she was lying down. I could feel no digital pulse while she was down. She "got up with a little difficulty the first time I asked her," but she seemed "sore in the right hip—maybe neuritis from the two hours of anesthesia" on her back, I speculated in her record. I gave her another 2 grams of Bute IV. She was walking and grazing very little in the round pen, so I turned her out in a larger pasture where she walked further and straighter, and she grazed better.

While neither grain nor lush pasture had caused Linda's acute laminitis, I normally would withhold both when treating any horse for acute laminitis. I believe both can compound laminitis regardless of the cause, but because Linda was not grazing vigorously, and she was not passing adequate manure easily, I let her have some very nice pasture while watching to be sure she did not overindulge herself. I wanted the good grass to stimulate her as she continued to recover from the traumatic delivery and anesthesia six days earlier. I never saw evidence of Linda passing any manure on Monday, but twice I examined her rectally and both times her rectum was full of soft manure. I noted a bone spur from a previous injury on the bottom of her sacrum, and the second time I evacuated her Monday I noted in the record that "the anterior half of her rectum had good tone and contractions, but the posterior half was flaccid and unresponsive." She was on her feet moving around the pasture about nine hours on Monday and walked pretty well when encouraged. We flushed her uterus in the pasture, and the discharge was quite clear. Her cervix was still wide open, and we gave her more SMZ-TMP orally twice. She also got 2 grams of Bute IV at noon and 8 cc of Banamine IM at 8:00 pm. She had lost interest in the pasture at 4:00 pm, so we put her back in the round pen and she immediately laid down in the sand.

My son got her up rather easily at 5:45 pm and I returned to check on her at 7:30 pm. The first thing I noticed when I examined her that evening was that her pulse was a very high 80 but her respiratory rate was normal at around 16. Her pulse had fluctuated all week at the hospital between 32 and 80, mostly in response to pain and drug relief I believed. Her respiratory rate seemed to jump up and down with the outside temperature. In checking her digital pulses, which were very hard to detect, I noticed she was much more sore on her right hind and did not want to lift her left hind foot. Standing behind her, I saw her right thigh was dramatically swollen. The thigh seemed to be about 50% bigger than the left thigh, the gaskin about 20% bigger, and the top of her right hock about 10% bigger than the left hind. Whatever was causing this sudden swelling seemed to be going from the thigh down the leg. I had specifically inspected her udder for any sign of mastitis just four hours earlier, and I can't believe I would have missed such dramatic thigh swelling as I was now seeing while looking at her udder.

I got up and rechecked Linda at 2:45 am Tuesday. She was standing quietly with an absolutely normal respiratory rate in the significantly cooler night air, but her pulse was now near 100 (it was too dark to check exactly against my watch). Even though she had probably been standing relatively still in the sand round pen most of the night, her front digital pulses were very soft, and I could not feel them in the hind fetlocks. She lifted both front feet for me the easiest since the laminitis had started, and she walked off easily when asked. We had indeed removed most of the inflammation and edema from her laminae, and blood was flowing easily there.

At 6:45 am Tuesday, her pulse had dropped to 60 and her temperature was 100.8 degrees, but the right hind thigh was even more swollen and very tight down to the hock. I gave her 10 cc Bute IV, 6 cc Lasix IM, 12 cc Dipyrone IM, and 12 SMZ-TMP tablets orally. A rectal exam at that time showed for the first time since she had arrived that her rectum was not impacted. Other than the swollen leg, I felt we were making substantial progress. The laminitis had turned around, and I expected she would need less Bute than the first two days.

When I reported the laminitis turn around and the further swelling of the leg to Carol, she asked me to consult with another vet at a hospital about 2 1/2 hours north of us. He felt the severe swelling in the leg was likely a perivaginal abscess from the foaling trauma a week earlier which was likely to come to a head, rupture, and drain in a couple days. I could see a softening about an inch lateral and two inches below the bottom of the vulva where that appeared to already be starting. He also recommended hot compresses, poultices, and higher levels of injectable antibiotics than the oral SMZ-TMP we had been using.

I agreed to nearly all of his suggestions, but Carol decided she needed to take the mare to his hospital. In spite of the severely swollen thigh, Linda walked to the trailer 100% better than she had walked off just 48 hours earlier. When she arrived at the next hospital, their evaluation determined that in addition to the thigh abscess, Linda had advanced peritonitis with little hope for recovery. She was euthanized prior to their treating her any further.

When Linda got into trouble with the severely contracted foal, there were no good options for removing the dead filly. Each of the three options, C-section, embryotomy, and manual repositioning, carried serious risk of complications. I don't know whether the same choices would be made the next time, and I do not criticize those choices. I have listed the chronology to show how sick Linda was while her laminitis was being reversed simply by keeping her out and moving, stopping the Ace, giving her the minimum effective dose of Bute (in this case 6 grams one day), and maybe a little more cold hosing. The point of this report is to add to the volume of case reports which make me believe that acute laminitis, in even the sickest and largest horses, can be reversed if you can restore adequate circulation before the hypoxic laminae lose their grip.

This would have tremendous implications for horses like Barbaro that may have eventually recovered from their fractures if the circulation had been maintained to their laminae. I read an online news report on Barbaro in mid-December of 2006 when many people were speculating when Barbaro might be released from the hospital. The reporter described how Barbaro would "come out of his stall each day gingerly testing his surgically repaired hind legs, now that it was too cold for his daily 20-minute outdoor grazing sessions." Toward the end of his 20-minute in-hospital walk, "Barbaro would again be confidently strutting like the proud champion he was." I could not disagree more. Even smart horses like Barbaro do not walk gingerly because they are being careful. They walk that way because their feet hurt from inadequate circulation while they are confined to their stall for 23 hours and 40 minutes a day. A month later, Barbaro's second bout of severe laminitis was announced as an unavoidable tragedy. I could not disagree more.

I had learned the hardest laminitis lesson of all in 1979 when I let myself be overruled by two excellent and nationally prominent hospital vets on Peter's very mild acute laminitis. They said, "It's absolutely not laminitis, it's navicular disease." They de-nerved Peter and a month later his coffin bones came through his soles without further warning, because I never realized he had been eating leaves off an oak tree which hung over his round pen. In 1989, I lost Jet to very mild laminitis which only showed itself when he came out of his stall first thing in the morning. I watched him jog fine on the track, but I never examined him, and he also had to be euthanized within a month, without being diagnosed or treated. I wrote up both these case reports over 15 years ago, but the journals consider them mere anecdotes and refuse to even consider publishing them, so others might learn from my worst mistakes. Experience can be the best teacher if we understand what is happening.

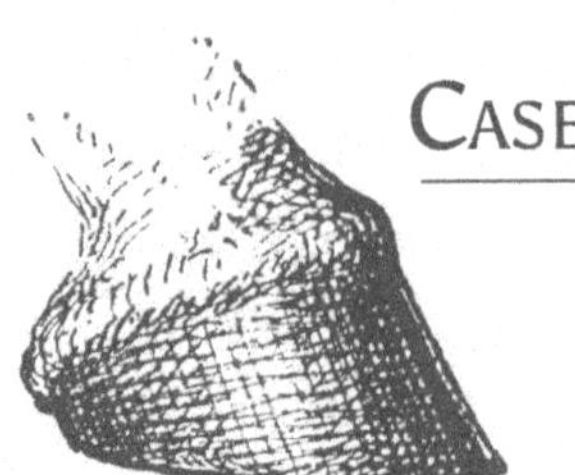

## Case Study

# "Nero"

*Saved From Hospital Treatment*

WHILE LILLIE INSISTED THAT NERO'S registration papers proved he was a pure Polish bred Arabian, I always felt his super friendly disposition, confidence, and conformation gave him much more of a Morgan horse appearance. For over ten years, he was a pleasure to work with every time I saw him. I would have been thrilled to have 100 more patients just like him.

I received Lillie's emergency call just after 5 pm on Friday, June 7, 1985. Nero was being kept by himself in a small barn and paddock and fed each morning by a high school boy not familiar with horses. When Lillie stopped to feed him after work, she saw that the barn was a mess. Nero had apparently gotten into his feed room the night before, but the boy did not realize the significance. He put Nero's regular morning feed out, closed the barn door, and went to school. By 5 pm, Nero was a little bloated and not interested in his evening feed.

I was already late for a dinner party that my wife and I were hosting for friends who were visiting for the weekend. Nevertheless, Nero was special to me, and I took the time for one more call before going home. Nero's colic was not severe, but he did have excessive gas, and the rectal exam, despite plenty of soft manure in his rectum, revealed a very firm pelvic flexure which is a common site of impactions. I gave him 12 cc of Dipyrone to relax his intestine, and 12 cc of Bute because of the danger of laminitis from both the possible impending impaction and the unknown quantity of grain he had helped himself to 18 hours earlier. Unfortunately for Nero, I had used the gallon of mineral oil I carried earlier in the day. It would have been very helpful for both the impending impaction and stopping endotoxins from the grain overload the night before. There was no time to go home and return. Since Nero was likely to need repeat visits over the weekend while I was scheduled hosting our visiting friends, I asked Lillie if she could take Nero to a hospital where they had live-in intern vets who could monitor Nero right through the weekend. Lillie understood my predicament and agreed to take Nero to the hospital.

Lillie called again on Saturday afternoon to update me on Nero's treatment at the hospital. First, she had not been able to find a trailer ride to the hospital until Saturday morning. After their exam that morning, he was given 5 cc Banamine, 1/2-gallon mineral oil, 32 oz. Pepto-Bismol, and 20 cc penicillin. He was eating hay and passing small piles of manure. He showed no foot pain, but they were going to check his digital pulse for possible laminitis every three or four hours, day and night through the weekend.

At 6 am Sunday, just about 47 hours after being found in the grain Friday morning, Nero showed his first sign of soreness in both front feet. At that time, he was given 2 grams of Bute paste, 20 cc of penicillin, and put back in his stall at the hospital. At 8 am Sunday, the other intern was able to feel the first rise in Nero's digital pulse pressure whereupon he was given 10 cc Banamine (on top of the 2 grams of Bute two hours earlier), 1-gallon mineral oil, and started on 10,000 units Heparin (a blood thinner) four times a day. In the 1980s, some researchers reported seeing small blood clots in the laminar vessels, so some professors were advising heparin for acute laminitis. I always believed the reported small blood clots of Disseminated Intravascular Coagulation or DIC were the result, not the cause of the poor circulation, so I was never tempted to use anticoagulants. Most other vets stopped using heparin also when they eventually saw no benefit from its use.

By 2:30 pm Sunday, Nero was "rocked back on his haunches, definitely painful." At 6 pm, the interns packed his front shoes level with plaster of Paris cast material. The idea was to prevent his coffin bone from rotating or sinking. I much prefer getting his shoes off and light walking on soft footing to prevent sinking or rotating by restoring optimum circulation as soon as possible. That is very hard to do if you insist on locking him in a stall. Nero was also given another 1 gallon of mineral oil and 500 mg of Banamine at 6 pm Sunday. The Heparin was continued through the night.

Early Monday morning, Nero was given another 500 mg of Banamine (a total of 20 cc, plus 2 grams Bute in past 24 hours.). He was taken out of his stall Monday morning and observed to be walking well on the straightaway but was "slightly sore turning." He still had a significant digital pulse and was started on oral aspirin powder.

Lillie had kept me informed of Nero's laminitis over the weekend. The hospital vets and interns were not at all optimistic that Nero would recover without significant rotation. She was also previously aware that I treated acute laminitis much differently than Nero was being treated at the hospital and with a much more optimistic prognosis if logical treatment is started early. Lillie decided to bring Nero home much to the dismay of the hospital vets who thought he was far too fragile for a trailer ride.

By coincidence, I happened to be driving by Nero's barn late Monday afternoon while Nero was being unloaded from the trailer. I stopped to look at him, and while I definitely did not agree with the hard cast material inside his shoes, he was walking extremely well in the road right off the trailer. He was doing so well we just put him in his stall and continued the treatment plan prescribed by the senior hospital vets, who had reviewed and approved his weekend treatment on Monday morning.

Lillie drove to the barn Tuesday morning to check Nero herself before going to work. She found him unable to move—definitely Grade IV acute laminitis 48 hours after his first sign of hoof pain Sunday morning. I was at his barn within 15 minutes and immediately gave him 12 cc of Bute and 8 cc of Lasix IV. I had to file off Nero's nail clinches with his feet on the ground. With extreme difficulty, I was able to get the first shoe and cast material off. The second was much easier as he now had a relatively reasonable foot to stand on. When both shoes were removed, he walked well enough to drop from Grade IV to Grade II within ten minutes.

Nero's water trough was in a sharp corner of his paddock where it was always a little muddy. We tied Nero in the corner and started hosing his feet. By the end of the day Nero had mud more than ankle deep. For the next month Lillie would put him in that mud three or four times a day. He was also given decreasing doses of Bute twice a day for most of the month—always at the minimum effective daily dose to keep him walking comfortably. I trimmed his front feet a couple times to keep his toes short for easier breakover, and his heels low for better frog pressure and heel expansion as he walked.

When I reviewed Nero's hospital records later that week, I noticed that his heel nerves had been blocked Monday afternoon in order to change the cast material inside his shoes just before Lillie had picked him up Monday. That made him look so much better than he really was at the time.

Other than the extreme mud treatment, Nero's month of recovery was quite uneventful. Nero was not a fat horse, but he did have an "easy keeper" metabolism with enough body fat to store, and then slowly release the endotoxins absorbed from the colic for nearly a month. By mid-July he had been off Bute and sound for over a week when Lillie resumed riding him barefoot. He had no other laminitis episodes in the ten years I cared for him.

I should warn here that some laminitis cases cannot tolerate so much mud and water. If the horse has too thin a sole and the coffin bone has already rotated, getting it too wet and soft can kill him. Knowing the difference requires daily observation and good judgment. Nero was one of the first, of five horses in this book, who responded far better to laminitis treatment at home than they had in the hospital.

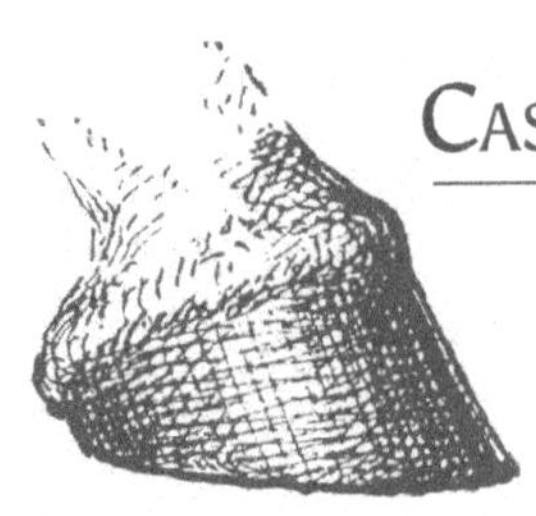

## Case Study

# "Sammy" and "Sunny"

### *Clover, Cresty Necks, and Colic Leading to Laminitis*

SAMMY AND SUNNY DO NOT have as slow a metabolism as the six previous horses, but I'm writing about them here because they shared a pasture with Rojo and both had unusual and educational laminitis attacks. At the time I was not the regular vet for Sammy, but his owner, Donna, called me when she realized he had laminitis, because she liked the advice I had given Rojo's owner better than the way her vet had previously been treating Rojo (pages 201-202).

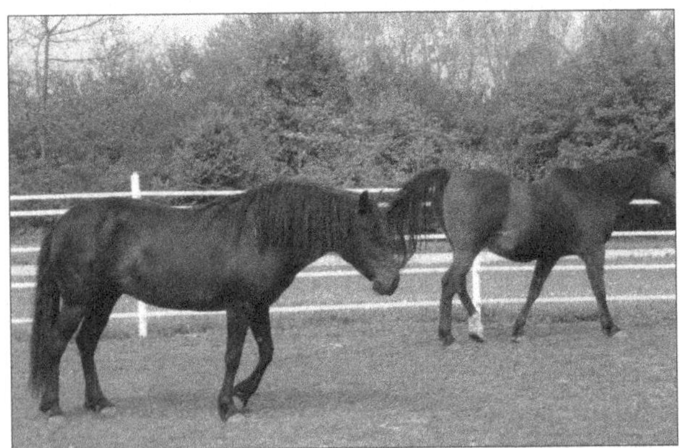

Sammy was a 20-year-old Arab gelding with excellent feet. He was significantly overweight and on the same pasture as Rojo, but he did not get his first acute laminitis attack until a couple years later. He had already had very obvious moderate laminitis pain for a couple days when Donna called me. I had her put him on a diet, using a grazing muzzle and gradually reducing doses of Bute. He was fine and off Bute within the week.

Sammy's second ever acute laminitis attack was nine years later, and he very nearly died of colic. He had a strangulated small intestine from rolling with a mesenteric lipoma on a stalk. Everything had to go perfectly that day, from Donna seeing the colic start, to me quickly making the diagnosis at the farm, then getting him to a hospital with an outstanding surgeon on duty, Dr. Christina Hewes. Sammy was on the surgery table less than two hours after the colic began. Most owners would not have invested the very substantial surgical and recovery expenses in a 28-year-old gelding with such poor survival odds after surgery (that required the removal of 35 feet of small intestine).

To her credit, Donna never balked at the expense or the poor odds. Sammy came through the major surgery amazingly well. He did have a nephro-splenic entrapment colic five weeks after the major surgery, which was quickly corrected with a second ride to the hospital, but no additional surgery. Then a few weeks later, he somehow suffered a cracked jawbone, which left him unable to chew his fine grass hay for a few weeks. Donna cut the fine hay for him with scissors until his jaw healed. Because he had lost so much of his intestine, the surgeon had him on a special prescription pellet.

Donna called me in December 2011, about nine months after the surgery because she thought he had a laminitis relapse. Now, Sammy had excellent feet and he suffered no damage whatsoever from his week with laminitis nine years earlier. He looked amazing, having gained all his weight back from before the major colic surgery, and a little extra weight. He had an easily detectable digital pulse in both front feet. He would limp turning in the barn aisle but walk fine on the straight away. Holding up a front foot for 30 seconds and then trotting him down the aisle would show an obvious lameness in the foot he had to stand on for 30 seconds.

I considered it barely Grade II acute laminitis and put him on just 2 grams of Bute for what I expected to be just a few days. I checked Donna's grass hay and found it was loaded with grass seeds. Since Donna was still cutting it for him with scissors, I asked her to cut the seeds out and give them to her other horse who had never had a laminitis attack.

Sammy's stable mate, Sunny, was much different. She was a six-year-old Peruvian Paso when Donna called me "to X-ray her feet." She lived in the same pasture as Sammy and Paso Rojo, but I was not their regular vet at the time. She wanted me to X-ray her horse's feet because the young mare would occasionally be lame in the pasture.

I wanted to see the lameness before X-raying her, but the mare would not trot a straight line on a lead rope (most Pasos don't trot). We turned her out in a square paddock, about 100 feet long on each side—about twice as big as a normal round pen, but with square corners. The "lame" mare would dart from corner to corner as quickly as a cutting horse, but with much higher hoof action. Probably about three or four times in the five minutes I watched her do this, she would dip a shoulder for a step or two like something might pinch her occasionally.

We brought her back in the barn. I could find absolutely no sore spot, from her toes to her nose. I X-rayed her feet as asked. The X-rays were as clean as the rest of her legs. I next received a call from Donna about three months later. She told me Sunny had laminitis for three months and nothing was stopping it. She had called her vet but was unable to stop it with Pergolide, Acepromazine, and short dosages of Bute. She was told, "Bute might cause an ulcer if given more than three days."

I felt the strong digital pulse that I had not felt three months earlier. Everyone knew the young mare was too fat, but the pasture was very short. When I walked out to check the pasture, there were huge patches of very short clover. This filly had thin lips and could eat the clover leaves closer to the ground; just as ponies can graze what a horse's lips are too thick to graze. I advised a grazing muzzle and the minimum effective dose of Bute as long as necessary, while monitoring the strength of the digital pulse. She recovered in a few weeks, without further damage.

Donna moved about 15 miles in 2011. Both Sammy and Sunny had repeated attacks of laminitis in the new pasture which had lots of clover. The clover in the paddock and pasture, with a very hard dry lot and mandatory stall time every night, unfortunately led to chronic laminitis in both Sammy and Sunny. Donna was an extremely generous client who loved her horses dearly, but she strongly resisted some of my advice. I repeatedly asked for a couple truckloads of sand to soften the dry lot, but it never happened. Both her horses developed almost allergic-like sensitivities to the clover, but she refused to kill it.

Donna spent extra for a "natural trimmer" who always resisted my requests for squared toes, to ease breakover and take the stress off the toe laminae. In the end, poor owner compliance was mostly responsible for the chronic laminitis in these two super-easy-keepers. Like the selections of stories elsewhere in this book, the failures are way over-represented here because of their teaching value. There were many, many, more successes which, by themselves, are of little teaching value.

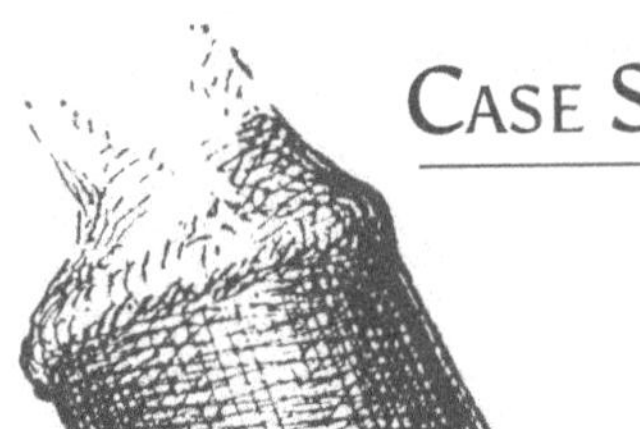

## Case Study

# "Bee Bee"

*Too Much of a Good Thing*

BEE BEE, A VERY SWEET older Arabian mare, was one of just 26 horses I had to euthanize because of laminitis/founder in my 42 years of practice in the same NW Chicago suburban area. Bee Bee was owned and lovingly cared for by Jerry, now sadly deceased himself. This was always one of my favorite visits because, after taking care of Jerry's horse business, he always enjoyed discussing nearly anything with me. A retired science teacher, he always had plenty of time to chat, and obviously missed his young students.

I was very surprised when Jerry first asked me to euthanize Bee Bee. He was upset because some days he would watch her struggle for several minutes before being able to get on her feet. Rather than euthanize her, I suggested a gram of Bute every day might ease her age-related arthritis pain and the resulting weakness in her hips. The one gram of Bute everyday kept Bee Bee comfortable enough that she made it through the winter and next summer very happily.

Eighteen months later (and I had visited Bee Bee and Jerry four times in the interim), Jerry called because her arthritis was getting much worse, and he had increased her Bute up to the maximum dose of 4 grams per day listed on the bottle. I went to again put Bee Bee to sleep, but this time I saw her problem was not the old arthritis, but severe laminitis. She had a very large and deep hoof ring almost an inch below each coronary band. Jerry was a bright, alert, well-educated man who personally took very good care of his horses, but he did not know how to differentiate acute laminitis from chronic arthritis which had been going on for several months. Jerry had provided Bee Bee all she could eat of extremely rich alfalfa. Jerry had increased the Bute as needed without realizing the alfalfa was the current problem, not her arthritic hips.

Instead of putting Bee Bee down, I squared her toes for easier breakover. We also took her off the alfalfa and continued the 4 grams of Bute. I told Jerry she needed to be out walking 24 hours because she was not getting enough circulation to the laminae in his stalls at night, standing on shavings over railroad tie floors.

We were too late in removing the source of the laminitis, and within a week Bee Bee's coffin bones dropped through her soles, and I had to put her down. She was one of just a few horses for which the free choice walking did not work; because the disease was so far advanced before it was diagnosed and properly treated. When the laminae are so stretched and inflamed, it can sometimes be too late for the treatment to work. After Bee Bee, I became more careful about prescribing even free choice walking after there is a lot of rotation and if the sole is relatively thin. I do not claim any special success in treating chronic laminitis with thin soles and major rotation or sinking. You must make the correct diagnosis early, treat the inflammation and edema causing vasocompression, not vasoconstriction, and identify and eliminate the cause. This works consistently before the damage has been done, but not after the rotation and sinking if the coffin bone is unstable.

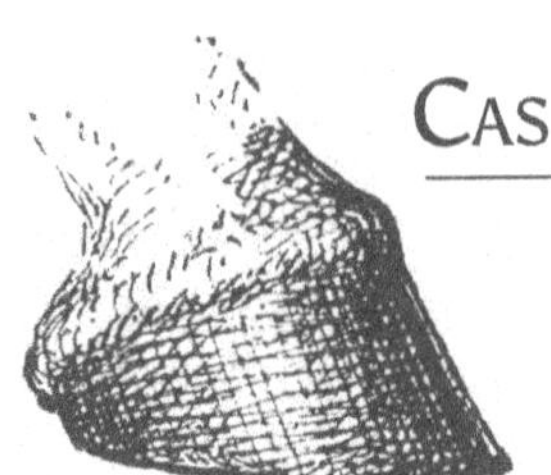

# Case Study

## "Joey"

### *The Most Severe Acute Laminitis from Fatal Vitamin K-3 Kidney Failure*

**AUTHOR'S NOTE:**

This story was written in 1985 with all the real names. Despite permission from all involved, the lawyers have insisted I change the names before publication. (38)

JOEY WON 19 OF HIS 20 races as a 2-year-old and was voted the National Champion 2-year-old Trotter in the 1970s. Not blessed with the soundness to match his heart, speed, and intelligence, Joey retired to stud after an injury plagued 3-year-old season, but he twice came back to win 13 more races in New York and Chicago in racing campaigns repeatedly interrupted by bone chips and two full breeding seasons. This was before digital radiography and arthroscopic surgery were developed.

In the early 1980s, I bred two very sound mares to Joey, hoping to get colts with his ability and their mothers' soundness. While Joey's rural Illinois farm was about 30 miles beyond my normal practice radius, I did occasionally make veterinary calls to his breeding farm. In early April 1984, I was one of seven different vets the owner consulted regarding blood showing up in now ten-year-old Joey's semen. He would typically be collected and several mares bred daily with artificial insemination. None of the seven vets had a solution for the blood in the semen issue other than to not breed the horse for a few weeks in the heart of the breeding season, or to give him some Vitamin K-3 to prevent the apparent testicular micro-hemorrhaging.

Early Friday morning, April 27, 1984, I received an unbelievable phone call from Joey's owner, Ken. He told me Joey had been at a hospital the past three days, and the vets there wanted to euthanize him due to irreversible kidney failure. My immediate response was, "Joey might be very sick and die, but you don't kill a once in a lifetime horse, unless the pain is uncontrollable." Joey had a giant heart, and we should not give up unless he had given up.

I told the owner I would call Dr. Phil, a personal friend/mentor, and the finest equine referral vet in the state of Illinois for about 40 years. If Dr. Phil had really given up on saving Joey, I told Ken we could bring him to my small farm in Barrington. Dr. Phil described Joey's rapid three day downward spiral at his hospital, and the inarguable blood tests. With his BUN and creatinine off the charts, Joey was clearly dying of kidney failure, and Dr. Phil simply told me, "If you want to bury him at home, you better get him before noon today, because he won't live any longer than that."

When Ken and I arrived at the clinic with my trailer that Friday morning, Joey was even worse than described over the phone. His face and head were blown up like a basketball. All four legs were severely swollen like stove pipes to above the knees and hocks, and he stood motionless in his stall hooked up to an IV drip trying to restart his failed kidneys. Joey's water bucket was filled to the brim, and he had not taken a sip in two days while on the IV fluids. Joey had last urinated a day earlier when he had reportedly passed a 12 inch by 3⁄4-inch blood clot in his urine. Most painful of all, when we tried to move him over in his stall, Joey had the most severe Grade IV acute laminitis.

Dr. Phil gave me the lab tests showing Joey's BUN at 205 and creatinine at 20.2, both of which were 10 to 20 times the normal range and very specific for kidney damage. Dr. Phil blocked Joey's digital heel nerves so we could walk him out of his stall and put him on the trailer. Before we left, Dr. Phil specifically cautioned me not to give him Bute or Lasix, because they are both "hard on the kidneys."

It was nearly noon when we arrived back at my small farm. The first thing I did after unloading Joey was give him 12 cc Bute IV and 10 cc Lasix IV against the very specific advice of the smartest vet I knew. They probably are "hard on the kidneys," but his kidneys were shut down, and the IV fluids had failed to stimulate them. Lasix was all I knew to restart his kidneys. Bute is crucial to get a horse with Grade IV acute laminitis moving, to restore circulation to his feet. I knew Joey was likely to die of the kidney failure, but I did not want him in the excruciating pain of severe untreated Grade IV acute laminitis.

Sure enough, within 15 minutes the Lasix caused Joey to urinate a blood clot as big as a 12" section of thick red cotton lead rope. We also started hosing his front feet and lower legs just outside the barn door. Before long Joey was standing in a mud puddle that wouldn't fully dry up for the next three years.

Joey initially got more sore, as the nerve blocks were starting to wear off, but after about an hour of constant cold hosing he started getting less painful and was moving around more as the edema was visibly leaving his legs, feet, and head. He still had very little interest in food or water, so we made a slurry of pellets in the blender, to which the non-drinking Ken had me add about six ounces of bourbon which a horseman had told him was good for sick horses. We fed him with a stomach tube. We started walking Joey in the small paddock that afternoon, and as is often the case with acute laminitis, after the first few steps Joey would walk much better. Getting the inflammation and edema out of his feet, and fresh blood into his feet, made an obvious improvement in his attitude.

While hosing Joey's feet and walking him all afternoon we had a lot of time to speculate on what might have caused the kidney failure. Ken was convinced it was the Vitamin K-3 he had given Joey two days before he went off feed, a week earlier. Like every other vet who had tried to imagine what could have caused the sudden and massive kidney damage, I dismissed the Vitamin K-3 as being a non-factor while I speculated about poisonous plants in his paddock or discarded antifreeze, leaking old batteries, or some other industrial toxins. Joey's paddock had been searched by another vet earlier in the week with no likely suspects. I also made a couple phone calls to human physician/clients exploring the possibility of doing some equine abdominal dialysis, but this was 1984 and nothing was available. Nevertheless, by late afternoon, Joey was doing so much better—walking the paddock on his own—that we went up to the house for dinner. When we returned about two hours later, Joey's attitude and comfort had regressed so much that one or both of us stayed constantly with him the rest of the night.

By 7:00 am Saturday morning, April 28th (after 19 hours of nearly constant hosing and walking, plus second doses of Bute and Lasixfurosemide), Joey showed no sign whatsoever of the severe laminitis the day before. All the swelling and edema was gone, and Joey was actually strutting and prancing around his new paddock, calling to my mares in the adjacent field. He looked, on the outside, like the proud champion he was, as the morning sun literally sparkled on his dappled spring coat. I had seen the horse probably 25 times the previous eight years, and he truly never looked better to me than he did after a full night of hosing his feet and grooming him.

Ken, a pessimist by nature, called his son in Iowa to report, "We're not out of the woods yet, but there's been a miracle." I really believed the horse looked like he had been raised from the dead and was in the height of his glory, but his kidneys were probably still not working right, so I took a blood sample that beautiful Saturday morning and sent it to the lab.

My wife had been out of town Friday, but both she and Ken's wife joined us on Saturday. In shifts, someone was always visiting with or grooming Joey all day Saturday in his new paddock. I left several times to call on other clients, but I was always just a page away in case he slipped backwards again. The constant familiar human companionship made a huge difference in the stallion's spirits and comfort.

My wife and I had a prior commitment for a friend's 50th birthday dinner Saturday evening which we wanted to cancel, but Ken and his wife insisted they would call us if Joey showed any sign of deterioration again. I had twice given Joey doses of Solu-Delta-Cortef when he seemed to be losing a little ground Friday evening and Saturday afternoon. I was afraid the short-acting steroid might be giving us a false sense of well-being without having cured anything.

We went to the dinner party around 5 pm, and about 8 pm Ken went up to the house for a glass of water. He sat down in a soft chair for "just a minute," but did not wake up until 10 pm. Ken immediately rushed back to the barn to check on his old friend and found Joey had collapsed and could not get up. When I arrived about 20 minutes later, Joey was toxic and disoriented. His circulation had collapsed, and he was dying of toxic shock.

As I put Joey to sleep, I could not help but think he had died the way he raced, giving everything he had way beyond what anyone had a right to expect of him. As long as one of us was present, he would not give up, or even show pain. Just before I euthanized him, I tapped on Joey's front feet with the hoof testers. The pain in his hooves, that was intolerable 36 hours earlier, was gone.

Since the cause of Joey's kidney failure was still a mystery, I did a full autopsy in the paddock with a light-but-steady rain falling after church Sunday morning. The pathology report a week later confirmed widespread renal necrosis (death of individual kidney cells). The blood tests we had taken Saturday morning when he looked so spectacular on the outside, came back on Monday with most chemistry values showing there was no question he had died of kidney failure (my only such case of kidney failure in 42 years of private practice).

Two weeks later, on May 15, 1984, the lead article on the cover of the *JAVMA* was "Vitamin K-3 induced renal toxicosis in the horse" (39). The history and blood tests of five private referral horses prior to 1983 (each with sudden kidney damage following Vitamin K-3 treatment at the racetrack for lung bleeding), followed by six experimental horses at Cornell University in 1983 matched Joey's case perfectly. Despite this article in the premier U.S. veterinary journal and repeated calls to the FDA's adverse drug reaction hotline, a year later this mislabeled and deadly drug was still on the market.

It took a million-dollar product liability lawsuit to get the mislabeled Vitamin K-3 off the market. Freedom of Information Act and trial discovery eventually showed that the FDA had approved a label with a 100-fold error in dosage. Someone had moved the decimal point the wrong way in converting pounds to kilograms years earlier, and no one at the drug manufacturer or the FDA had caught the simple math error. The million dollar plus settlement in this case also acknowledged that future stud fees could be considered in addition to market value in determining damages.

However, the main point of this sad story about a great horse's end, is that no matter how sick a horse is—even 36 hours beyond when he should have died from total kidney failure—the very most severe case of acute laminitis can be totally reversed if you can restore optimum blood flow by reducing inflammation and edema in the feet, and letting the horse walk unshod on soft ground.

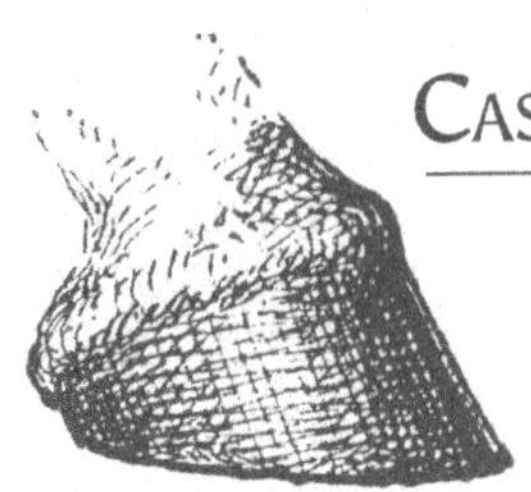

## Case Study

# "Amber"

### *Diagnosing Acute Laminitis Can Be Difficult After 8 Grams of Bute*

AMBER WAS A 9-YEAR-OLD Irish Draft mare in the fall of 2009. She stood 17.1 hands and easily maintained her 1,400-pound weight on just three flakes of hay twice a day.

I had only seen Amber twice before October 15, 2009. In the spring of 2009, she was among the 12 horses I had been asked to vaccinate for the first time for a new client. The owner, Jane, mentioned that Amber had colic surgery a few months earlier, but she looked to be fully recovered, and we moved on to the next horse rather quickly.

When I returned to the farm on September 30th for the fall rhino-flu booster shots, Jane mentioned Amber was prone to hoof abscesses, and she seemed to be having trouble recently. She was not dead lame, but it was fairly easy to see she was more tender on her right front foot. With the aid of hoof testers, I was easily able to locate and open a half inch deep hole in the white line at the toe of her right front sole. Unlike a typical abscess, no liquid pus was released, but a significant amount of necrotic white line was removed, and the resulting hole filled with iodine and cotton, which Jane cleaned and changed daily for the next two weeks. Jane next called on October 15 to report that Amber had been better right after we had cleaned out her right front toe, but she now seemed bothered by abscesses in the other foot! She said she was just not moving right and spending more time lying down. Sometimes she would rock back on her haunches, then other times she would come "charging up for her feed." The owner's description over the phone that it was now both front feet made me think this could be laminitis. I felt I needed to see her that day. Jane worked days and thought it would be fine to wait until the weekend.

I persisted and Jane made arrangements to leave work early that same afternoon, so I could see Amber just a couple hours after she had called. I do not like to let possible laminitis cases wait for a convenient appointment for both the owner and the vet. Laminar damage can happen quickly while waiting days, or even overnight, for the appointment.

Jane called again while I was on my way to her farm, because I had misunderstood the agreed upon hour, and I was late. I asked her if Amber was in her stall or the pasture. She said she was in the indoor arena. I asked her to put her in the stall until I would arrive in about 15 more minutes. I asked for this stall confinement in case she had very mild laminitis. It would then be easier to feel a digital pulse after she had been in the stall for a while.

When I arrived, I reached down to feel Amber's digital pulse before we brought her out of the stall. I had a very hard time feeling the pulse behind her left front fetlock, and I could not feel a pulse at all behind her right front. Jane wanted me to show her how to feel the pulse, but I hesitated, because I could barely find one myself. When there is a significant pulse, I always teach the owner to feel it, because for me it is key to monitoring progress and treatment of laminitis. To my surprise, Jane felt the pulse very quickly behind Amber's left front fetlock, but she was also unable to feel a pulse behind the right front hoof.

We then brought Amber into the aisle. She readily picked up each front foot for me, but she constantly tried to pull them away from me as I cleaned them and tried to go around each sole with the hoof testers. I presumed this was just bad manners in a very large, partially broke, and anxious horse who was more interested in rejoining the other horses. I was unable to find any tender spots with the hoof testers to explore for an abscess. The fact that she readily picked up each front foot made it less likely that she had a significant abscess in the foot she was left to stand on.

Next, I asked Jane to lead her up and down the aisle while I watched carefully for any increased pain as she pivoted and turned. The large mare was still distracted by her pasture mates, but I saw no increased pain when she pivoted in the aisle. I was having a hard time determining whether the soreness and unevenness Jane had called me about could be due to very small abscesses or very mild laminitis. Amber was kept outside 24/7, and Jane again mentioned that while she had seen her lying down more than usual, and moving unevenly, there would be times when she would come "charging up to the barn" like nothing at all was bothering her.

There was no straight, flat, hard surface near the barn to watch the big mare trot off; so I finally told Jane that I thought, while she may have been tender in both front feet alternately because of gravel and other debris in the barnyard, I really suspected she had a very mild case of laminitis. I was having a hard time confirming the diagnosis because she was outside 24/7 and a very fidgety horse. The 15 minutes she was in the stall, she was back and forth the whole time wondering why she could not rejoin the others. I believed this constant movement kept enough fresh blood flowing to her laminae to normalize her digital pulse pressure. Or she may have been a horse with an unusually high pain threshold. I really did not know the horse very well.

I suggested one gram of Bute per day for a couple days to see if that improved her gait in the pasture. Amazingly, only then did Jane tell me she had given Annie 4 grams of Bute the night before and 4 more grams that morning before she left for work. I should have asked for this bit of extremely important history at the beginning of the exam. Even if I did not ask, the owner should have told me. Eight grams of Bute in less than 24 hours, even for a very large mare, totally changed my interpretation of what I had seen. She absolutely had significant acute laminitis, and Jane having seen her "rock back on her haunches" prior to giving the Bute made more sense now. The periodic "charging up to the barn" after having seen her obviously uncomfortable and lying down more that week is an unusual response. I've only seen hard running in four other laminitis patients, but I have also seen it in very sore racehorses a few times. An occasional racehorse feels better "running through the pain."

Next, we had to check Amber's hay. The hay was a very good mix of mostly grass, but there was also a significant amount of clover and alfalfa in the hay. It was obviously second cutting with some of the grasses having gone to seed, effectively adding protein to the mostly grass hay. I suggested that Jane shake out the hay for Amber in the aisle, then pick the stems off the top to feed her and give the leaves and seeds to another horse who could use a little extra.

We then checked her turnout area. Because she was an easy keeper, who had colic surgery nine months earlier, Amber was kept and fed separately from the other 11 horses in several different paddock groupings. Amber's private paddock was all dirt, or mud if it rained, which was the case about 25 of 31 days in October 2009. There were a few unidentified weeds growing in the paddock alongside the barn, a couple of which Amber had eaten from, and the others she had ignored. It can be hard to guess what a horse on a strict diet will decide is suitable to eat. There was also a young maple tree about five feet over a fence, with a hot wire on top of the fence, apparently out of reach. The tree was changing colors that week from green to red. Red maples can be deadly to horses, especially if they eat the leaves as they are wilting after a branch is cut, or comes down in a storm. There was no obvious indication Amber had eaten from that tree.

I told Jane that I would e-mail her a number of my case reports on laminitis, so that she might get a better understanding of my laminitis theory and treatment plans. Early the next morning I sent her about six case reports, plus two discussions on the danger of Bute toxicity.

I did not hear from Jane over the weekend, so I presumed Amber was coming along well on the minimum effective dose of Bute we discussed. I again e-mailed Jane at work on Tuesday morning to ask about Amber's progress. Jane responded that Amber was making steady daily progress from 60% sound the day before I saw her to "65%, 70%, 75%, 80%, and now 85% sound on 2 grams of Bute." I responded that I've never been able to tell the difference between 70% and 75% sound, but I appreciated the point that Amber was making steady observable progress and the Bute was being appropriately decreased.

I only saw Amber two more times for vaccinations in the spring and fall 2010. The laminitis soreness which was so hard for me to diagnose in 2009 reportedly resolved within a week of the hay being shaken out, along with successively lower doses of Bute. There was no visible damage to her feet. I wrote up this case because it was so hard to make the laminitis diagnosis after 8 grams of Bute. Please tell your vet if your horse is on Bute while he is doing a lameness exam!

# ~SECTION VII~

## TYPICAL CASES

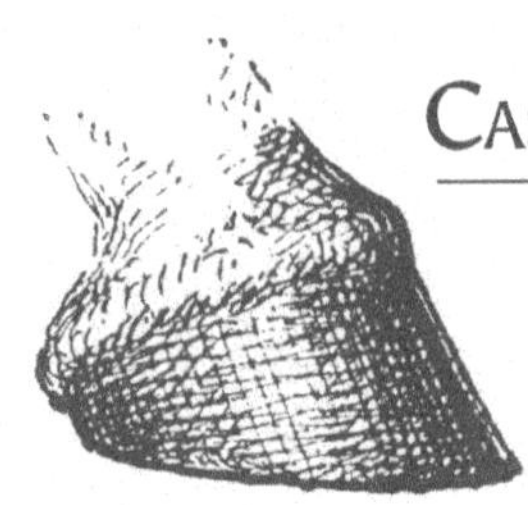

## Case Study

# "Black Tie Cody"

### *Grade III Laminitis to the Show Ring in 7 Days*

CODY WAS A SOUND, PLEASANT, well-trained, and attractive black, 13-year-old QH gelding when Debbie purchased him for her first horse on February 19, 2003. His three-day bout with Grade III acute laminitis over Labor Day weekend 2003 is presented here, not because of anything unusual or extreme about the case. Rather it represents the simplicity of laminitis, and the most typical presentation and response to treatment I have seen in private practice.

While this case's simplicity is typical of at least 20–30% of the 1,200 plus cases I have treated, it exposes a number of the myths I have seen written about laminitis the past 42 years, while I have been treating acute laminitis in my suburban/rural, backyard/farm equine practice. Unlike the other acute laminitis cases I have written up, which tend to come from the extreme ends of the spectrum, either so mild that their disease was missed by several experienced veterinarians, or so severe, fat, or sick that they seemed to have no hope. Cody's case was very straight forward.

Labor Day weekend 2003 happened to be my 25th wedding anniversary, and my wife and I had the long holiday weekend packed with six different celebrations with my family, her family, our friends, and our three children each starting a new school soccer or field hockey season that weekend. While I had scheduled no appointments for the long weekend, I was on call 24/7 for emergencies, as always.

Debbie called about Cody Saturday morning while I was at my daughter's field hockey tournament. She said Cody had been shod Friday after work, and then moved to her cousin's house Friday evening because she wasn't happy with her previous boarding situation. Her cousin called Debbie on Saturday morning to tell her Cody was not walking right, was lying down too much, and she needed to get a vet to see him. From her description, I couldn't tell if Cody was colicky, shod with a close nail, or had laminitis. Debbie had no prior experience with any of the conditions I was considering, and because she hadn't seen Cody that morning, she couldn't answer my questions about whether he would eat grass, if he was pawing or sweating, if he seemed more sore in just one foot, or if he walked better after his first few steps. She did assure me that he was not fat and he had no recent diet change or anything unusual to eat.

Because I couldn't be sure from Debbie's answers what the problem was, I asked to have her cousin call me. A couple minutes later her cousin Laura assured me that Cody's appetite was fine, he was not pawing or sweating, and he seemed "sore all over" not just one foot, however both front feet seemed to hurt the worst. I was confident he had acute laminitis, despite Laura also assuring me he was not at all fat, but actually rather lean.

Laura, with a half dozen horses at her home, had some Bute on hand and was familiar with laminitis. I asked her to give Cody 2 grams of Bute and find an area where she could make a mess running a cold hose on his feet. Then I asked her to call me back in two hours when the field hockey tournament would be over and I could decide, depending on Cody's response to the Bute and cold water hosing, whether my wife, daughter, and I could meet about fifteen of our relatives for a planned picnic lunch before my son's 3:00 soccer game, or if I needed to go home right away for my vet truck to see Cody.

Laura called back in an hour and a half to report that Cody was about 80% better, walking pretty well and eating just fine. She and Debbie were willing to alternately hose his feet and turn him out in the sand arena the rest of the afternoon until my son's soccer game was over. After the lunch and ten minutes into the soccer game, I had two more calls that needed to be seen Saturday afternoon before our evening party.

After finishing with the two calls, I saw Cody at 5:00 pm. I had only seen Cody and Debbie twice before (at his pre-purchase exam and once for a vaccination and minor thrush). He was at least 50 pounds lighter from a summer on pasture battling the flies with a half dozen other horses and competing for too little grass after a month's drought. While Debbie and Laura insisted he was much better than he had been prior to the Bute and cold hosing, he still had an easily detectable digital pulse in both front feet. He was still short-strided, especially the first few steps after standing a couple minutes. He also hurt noticeably to turn at a walk when pivoting on his front feet applied torque to the still sensitive laminae.

I showed both ladies how to feel Cody's digital pulse over the base of his fetlock. The strength of the digital pulse is one of my key signs of laminitis, the response to treatment, and the level of Bute still needed to arrest the inflammation within the feet.

Normally, I would remove the shoes, square the toes, and lower the heels to ease breakover and increase frog pressure and hoof flexibility for a case of laminitis. However, Cody was the exception to my rule, since he had just been reset the night before with a pair of rubber, wide-webbed, frog bar shoes. These were the most flexible shoes I've ever seen. The nails were set well forward so as not to interfere with heel expansion. And the frog and bar sections, along with the 1-inch-wide web, distributed the ground pressure over a large area of the sole, bars, frog, heel, and hoof wall. Because his foot was freshly trimmed flat for the shoeing, Cody would have been more sore if I had removed his shoes, thus aggravating the inflammation within the hoof rather than alleviating it.

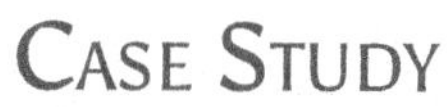

# Case Study

## "Alfresca," "Domingo," and "Tuffy"

### *Three 2007 Spring Pasture, First-Time Acute Laminitis Cases—Two Cures and One Sudden Death*

I HAVE NOT PERSONALLY CONDUCTED double-blind, controlled studies to support my views on the causes and best treatment of laminitis. However, using actual counts over the most recent 24 years, I conservatively estimate that I have diagnosed and treated over 1,200 laminitis cases in my 42 years in the same private NW suburban Chicago equine practice. Each of these cases individually is considered merely an anecdote by the medical journal editors who do not consider what I have observed and learned "scientifically valid."

Contrary to the oft-quoted opinion of most researchers, in my practice there is rarely permanent clinical damage at the time lameness is first seen. My patients have never died of laminitis "due to the mysterious nature of the disease." All 26 horses I euthanized due to laminitis had specific increased risks and/or direct causes to start the disease. In every euthanasia case I saw, somebody "dropped the ball" in treatment—either me, the owner, the trainer, the barn manager, another vet, and two very good farriers. Using bad advice of the day, one farrier put severe 18-degree wedge pads on a laminitis flare-up, to relieve tendon pull, without any medical treatment or diet changes. Another very good farrier admitted, after I had to euthanize one of his client's horses, that the horse had been dramatically difficult at its last shoeing. It can be very difficult for a horse with acute laminitis to stand on one front foot for the farrier. She was not foundered yet, so her sole looked normal to the farrier, but two weeks later when the vet was called, the horse was foundered beyond repair. You have to recognize the acute laminitis whether the pain is mild or severe. Mild is harder to diagnose, but you have a longer window of opportunity; severe cases can go very fast. In eight ponies and minis of my over 1,200 cases (including Tuffy in this story), slight overdoses of Bute, or individual hypersensitivity to the drug might have killed the ponies.

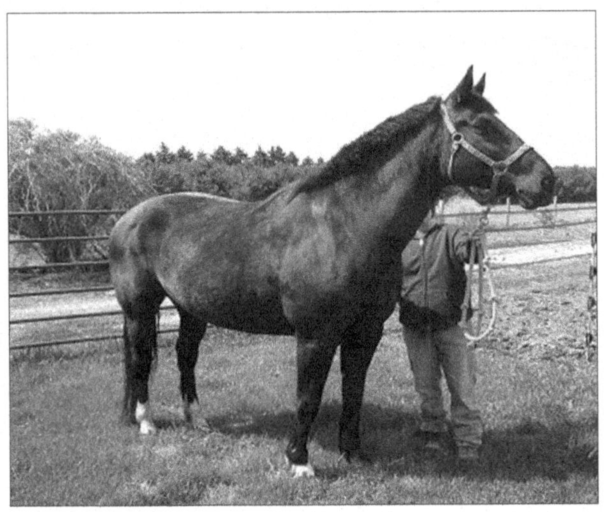

*Alfresca*

Alfresca, a Warm Blood X Percheron, Domingo, a large Tennessee Walker, and Tuffy, the Mini, are three cases from 2007 which illustrate how simply severe cases can be cured, and how far I sometimes had to go to be the horse's advocate. I was always aware of the real risk of losing the client to a more tactful and politically correct veterinarian. I had little interest in the lifetime care of founder complications, which can be a very lucrative practice for some veterinarians. Every spring as I made the rounds of my patients for the annual vaccinations, Coggins tests, deworming, teeth floating, and sheath cleaning, I had to warn a few clients that their horses had gotten dangerously obese over the winter and were at high risk of serious laminitis as the pastures turned green. This was not something I would mention casually in passing. Some people like their horses fat, and my warnings could be as rude and obnoxious as telling the person themselves to lose weight. Domingo, Alfresca, and Tuffy were represented by four very different owner/clients, who each got my sternest "in their face" lectures on April 6, May 1, and May 15, 2007, respectively. Within a month of the warnings both Domingo and Alfresca, easily 150 to 200 pounds overweight, had their first ever bouts of severe Grade IV laminitis from lush spring pasture. Tuffy, a Minature horse I had known about eight years, experienced his first bout of acute Grade II laminitis as I was lecturing his owners, who had only called for the spring shots and Coggins tests. Each horse responded very well to treatment and management changes, but their stories are told here to illustrate what I had to do every spring to save horses from a lifetime of founder, and in Tuffy's case the double-edged sword of treatment may have killed him.

Domingo and Alfresca continue as very sound horses ten years later. Domingo's owner was a client all 42 years of my private equine practice. She had boarded her horses since high school with neighbors, friends, small farms, and finally a small boarding stable with daily pasture turnout. In all the years I've known the owner, I'll call her Sally, she had never before had to deal with laminitis. This professional lady was one of my most intelligent and best-educated clients. Unlike many horse owners, she kept her horses for the rest of their lives. Her first two horses died in their mid-30s.

I was called for Domingo's acute laminitis on May 8, 2007, 32 days after he had a throbbing pulse in all four feet and great pain all around when forced to walk. I immediately gave the 1,350-pound Tennessee Walker gelding 12 cc Bute IV and 6 cc Lasix IV. The anti-inflammatory, diuretic, and light walking relieved his pain as fresh blood returned to his laminae. Then I trimmed back his front toes and lowered his front heels for easier breakover and better frog support. We put him in a small dirt paddock and started hosing his feet by the water tub. No soft sand arena was available, so he was confined to the small paddock with a run-in shed 24/7 for the next two months. He was given two flakes of grass hay three times a day and started on 2 grams of Bute paste twice a day. The Bute was to be reduced to the minimum effective daily dose as he improved. Due to his obesity, I expected it to be about six weeks before all the endotoxins triggered by the spring pasture would be released from his fat cells, especially in the crest of his stiff neck.

He recovered uneventfully, receiving in divided doses 4 grams of Bute for three or four days, then 3 grams per day for about another week, then 2 grams per day for a couple more weeks, and 1 gram per day for the final three to four weeks. That was a total of 80 to 90 grams of Bute over six to seven weeks before he was absolutely sound off medications. I looked at him over the fence two or three times when I was at the farm or driving by to see him losing weight and progressing on schedule, but I was only called back to check his progress once during the course of his laminitis. I never X-rayed his large, well-shaped feet and certainly saw no need to do the venograms or use the therapeutic shoes currently being recommended by the national experts. He lost about 150 pounds during his uneventful recovery and looked quite good by early July. However, he did recover with a slight new separation at each front toe white line and he developed a small abscess in each front toe on July 20 and July 28, which were opened and drained in one visit each. Sally and the stable management kept his feet wrapped in diapers containing iodine and Epsom salts, secured with duct tape, for at least two weeks after he was again sound to give the abscesses a chance to regrow healthy sole from the inside out.

Domingo was sound for a month, before coming up sore again on September 1st. He had rejoined the others on pasture in mid-August, wearing a grazing muzzle to limit the amount he could eat. Unfortunately, it rained about ten of the first twelve days Domingo was back on pasture, and we got a second rapid growth of lush pasture. The September 1st soreness turned out to be due about 25% to a mild relapse of the laminitis from too much clover through the grazing muzzle, and 75% to plugging of one of the abscess holes in the toe with dirt and tiny gravel. We treated the laminitis flare-up with a few days of Bute, used duct tape to reduce the size of the grazing muzzle hole by 50%, and packed the cleaned-out abscess hole with iodine and a cotton ball, then layered duct tape over the hoof.

Domingo's serious laminitis episode sensitized him to lush pasture. In subsequent years he wore the grazing muzzle on pasture and received no alfalfa, clover hay, or grain until a rib was visible on him. After the annoying abscesses, he was absolutely fine to resume his trail rides with no drugs and standard shoeing or barefoot if he could avoid gravel. The next nine years Domingo had only one additional brief bout of laminitis.

Alfresca's owner was a newer client I'll call Jane, who used to show dressage horses as a younger adult. She bought a small farm near me and kept her two under-worked and over-fed horses in her 6-acre backyard stable and pasture, with two other huge ex-dressage Warmbloods. She was the personal caretaker/pamperer of the four giant retirees.

Alfresca, a 1,700-pound 3⁄4 Warm Blood X 1⁄4 Percheron mare normally came in for dinner every evening, but she would not come in on May 29th at 6:00 pm. When her owner went out to get her, she wouldn't move. Jane called my cell phone in a mild panic and described her predicament. I was out to a very nice restaurant for my wife's birthday party when I received the call for Alfresca's laminitis. I was expecting this since I had met this overweight horse, and I asked if she could feel a pulse at the back off her fetlock. She quickly said, "Yes." I told her from my dinner table that Alfresca had acute laminitis, and to get some help forcing her to walk, which should help her get a little better. Then hose her feet with cold water, give her 3 grams of Bute, which she had in her stable, and let her wander in a dirt paddock overnight with no grain and well-shaken hay, to get most of the alfalfa and clover leaves out. I told Jane I would be out early the next morning to check her, but I also asked her to call me back if Alfresca did not get significantly better shortly.

The dinner party ended earlier than I expected, and not hearing back from Jane, I felt guilty and decided to drive about ten miles to her farm and check the mare while there was still some summer daylight. I arrived about 8:00 pm, expecting to find them hosing the mare's feet, but instead learned from Jane's daughter that they had just left for an equine hospital with the mare on the trailer. After I had told Jane her mare had laminitis, she had called another daughter who is a trainer and assistant manager at another stable. The second daughter told her mother she had to get the mare to the hospital ASAP. The second daughter had brought her farm's rig over to pick up her mother's mare, who was indeed moving significantly better after the Bute, some walking, and hosing.

I then called Jane on her cell phone and told her that 50% of horses with laminitis in hospitals end up dead, whereas only 5% on farms have to be euthanized. I expected Alfresca to be absolutely fine if she brought her back home. I honestly was more concerned that the very large mare would do very poorly with laminitis treated in a hospital stall, than I was worried about any loss of revenue. I would send many horses to the hospital. If the mare had colic or a nasty wound, I would have been thrilled they had already decided to take her to the hospital. I could then rejoin my wife's birthday party.

They turned the rig around and had her back to the farm in about 20 minutes. Alfresca walked off the trailer obviously sore, but Jane insisted she had been "much, much worse" earlier. I understood, but she and her daughter, the young trainer, said the Bute must be killing her pain. I had to explain that while Bute is a pain killer, much more importantly it is an anti-inflammatory drug, which along with the hosing and walking relieves enough of the swelling to allow fresh blood to return to the stressed and painful laminae. It is the fresh blood that makes all the difference. The drugs simply help us get it past the swollen tissues.

Alfresca still had an easily palpable increased digital pulse pressure in all four feet. I explained the strength of that pulse was a very important guide to how much Bute or hosing the mare needed as her recovery progressed over the next six to eight weeks due to her obesity. Alfresca had very large round feet, but there was no excess toe or heel to trim. Her sole was not as concave as I would have liked. My only additional treatment was 6 cc Lasix, a diuretic, to help with her laminar edema.

My most difficult task was convincing Jane to leave Alfresca out 24/7. The mare had never spent the night under the stars since she had owned her. The owner was absolutely certain that if insects, coyotes, rain, or lightning didn't kill her 1,700-pound mare, then she would run through the fence in a panic in the middle of the night. I always insist on the minimum amount of stall time because I know a walking horse, on properly trimmed feet, gets better circulation to his feet than a stall-bound horse, and fresh blood is the most important treatment for acute laminitis.

Alfresca's recovery was a bit longer, but even less eventful than Domingo's. I was only called back to recheck her and deliver more Bute paste three times. She had a larger and softer loam paddock, which allowed her more room to roam than Domingo, and she was a naturally easier horse to chase off than the gelding. A clap of the hands or wave of the arms and she would take off rearing and kicking. I don't ask for that very often, but it was a good way to gauge her recovery progress and the level of Bute needed. She received about 100 grams of Bute over eight weeks, just slightly more than the smaller Domingo, but she recovered without any separation or abscess.

After I had not heard from Alfresca's owner in over a month, she called on August 10th asking me to check the mare's insulin level. She could still find a digital pulse some mornings after she had had no Bute for three or four days. Jane would then give Alfresca 1 gram of Bute, and the pulse would be gone for several days before coming back again. The mare had not lost much weight, and Jane's daughter felt that since it had been ten weeks there must be another problem. I was anxious to recheck the mare's current condition and agreed to discuss the need for the requested blood tests.

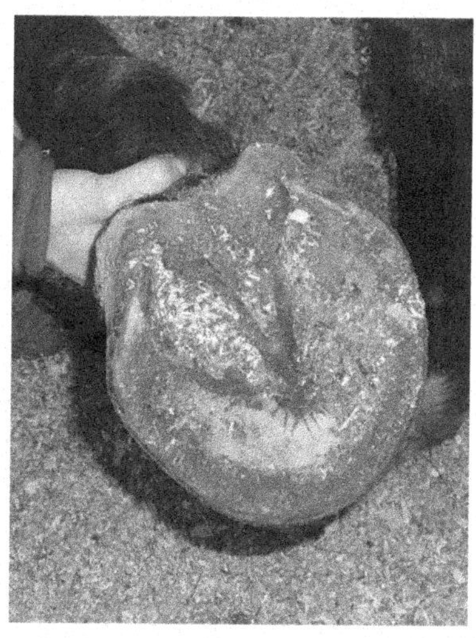

*Alfresca's Left Front Sole*

When I saw Alfresca on August 10th she looked like she may have lost only 20 or 30 pounds of the 200 pounds I wanted her to lose. Jane had given her 1 gram of Bute that morning, because she did have a pulse when she came out of her stall. I asked why she was in the stall overnight and learned she had only stayed out all night most of the first two weeks. Jane then resumed keeping her in every night because the horse was "happier in the barn at night with her friends." The owner readily admitted that she would be sorer going out in the morning, but then seemed fine all day in the dirt lot, or on pasture three hours wearing a muzzle. She was going out on the pasture with the muzzle every day, because, again, the horse was "happier when she was with her friends."

I heard nothing more until September 20th when Jane again called to report that Alfresca would be fine with no Bute and no detectable digital pulse for about eight or ten days. Then the pulse would suddenly reappear either when she came in from pasture, or before she was turned out in the morning. Jane would then give her 1 gram of Bute for a day or two and she would be fine for a week or ten days before she'd find the pulse again.

I congratulated Jane on her diligence for checking her mare's pulse at least twice a day. I have no doubt that if she were not so diligent in finding the pulse this mare would have already rotated. Despite wearing the muzzle in the pasture, Jane admitted she still had lost less than 50 pounds in almost four months.

If Jane were more concerned with her mare's health than her happiness, Alfresca would have lost much more weight and the laminitis would have been gone weeks earlier. Alfresca remained at very high risk of laminitis relapses because her owner insisted on putting her in a small 12' x 12' stall every night and refused to treat the mare's obesity seriously.

## AUTHOR'S NOTE:

After writing this article and giving it to Jane for review, she finally did get serious about Alfresca's weight. The next spring, she was at least 100 pounds lighter. She held that weight the next eight years and looks excellent today at 1,600 pounds rather than 1,700! She still stays in every night but has never had another laminitis bout. Alfresca's laminitis lingered most of a year because she lost weight very slowly and her owner could never bear to leave her outside 24/7. After she finally did lose her excess fat, she has remained Bute free the past nine years, and her feet and body look excellent today.

Tuffy, the Mini, suffered his only two bouts of laminitis in 2007. The Mini's owners were always difficult for me to communicate with effectively and recently retired. While Rick tried hard to understand and do what was necessary, his wife had an excuse for every suggestion I'd offer to change their pasture situation. I'd often have to think of five different ways to tell them the same thing before they seemed to grasp the seriousness of my suggestions. Actually, most clients do not listen to horse keeping suggestions very well, until their horses are in serious pain.

Tuffy's owners, who already had four horses in their 3-acre backyard stable, won the Mini weanling in a raffle at a horse expo in 1998. They raised him in a separate small lot from their four riding horses. He was always an obnoxious and poorly mannered handful for me to vaccinate. One of their mares died in 2006, and they sold two of the other horses in anticipation of their 2007 retirement to move to a warmer climate. Tuffy and the remaining Appaloosa gelding had become new best friends over the winter. And from his huge weight increase, it was clear that they were now being fed together and sharing the same pasture which was loaded with clover. As I vaccinated Tuffy on May 15th, I gave them my toughest laminitis lecture and the wife replied with excuses why they could not keep Tuffy off the clover and feed them separately. I was losing my argument for separate feedings when I suddenly realized that Tuffy was much better behaved than he had ever been. I reached down and easily felt the increased digital pulse pressure of acute laminitis. I asked Rick to lead Tuffy away and make a tight U-turn to bring him back. On turning Tuffy limped noticeably. I used hoof testers and Tuffy was tender at both front toes. He already had Grade II laminitis as we were speaking, but none of us had noticed.

I gave Tuffy just 1 gram of Bute paste and left the other 11 grams in the tube. I told the owners to give the minimum effective daily dose, which would probably be 1⁄2 to 1 gram most days, or maybe none if he was really moving well. I demanded that he go back in his separate small lot and be fed only grass hay.

The owners' only request over the next 2 1⁄2 months was to buy a second tube of Bute without a visit to recheck Tuffy. But on Wednesday Aug. 8, 2007, their neighbor called. Rosie, a very responsible and experienced high school girl was caring for Tuffy and the Appaloosa while the owners were out of town for a week. Tuffy was again sharing the clover-laden pasture with the larger horse, possibly to make it easier for Rosie. Tuffy had indeed lost a little weight and been off Bute and sound for most of two months. But it had rained nearly every day the first week of August, and the pasture that had been relatively dormant through a dry July, was now growing rapidly. When Rosie arrived to check the horses her second morning, Tuffy wouldn't move without being forced, and then limped very badly on both front feet. Rosie knew right away this was a severe laminitis emergency, and she had me there within the hour. We again gave Tuffy 1 gram of Bute paste, trimmed his heels a little (unlike most Minis, Tuffy had a great wide heel). Since they had no sand arena Rosie offered to take him home to her sand arena, a quarter mile up the road, after we tranquilized the Appy who had never been left alone before. Again, I left the rest of the 12-gram tube of Bute paste and told Rosie to give the minimum effective daily dose—not more than 1 gram per day.

I spoke with the owners by phone, who offered to cut their trip short and return home that day. I assured them that their neighbor was very capable and had already taken Tuffy to her house where she could hose his feet and leave him in her sand arena 24/7. Rosie also brought the Appaloosa to her home and put him in the sand arena with Tuffy. The next day she reported by phone that Tuffy, who could hardly move on Wednesday, was walking "much better." I did not need to recheck him. Four days later Rosie called on Sunday morning after church and said Tuffy was acting "very strange." I asked when the owners were returning, and she said they had gotten back late Saturday night. They had been to see Tuffy earlier Sunday morning, and all looked well to them. Since the owners were home, I asked the girl to have them come back to see Tuffy again. Then they should call me before deciding if I needed to make a Sunday emergency call.

The owners called and said Tuffy was absolutely fine earlier that morning, but was now in real trouble—not colic, but "just bad." I had one other Sunday emergency visit to stop by first, and the wife called again on my cell to tell me to hurry because the Mini "was dying." I arrived about 30 minutes later to find

Rosie's father blowing in Tuffy's nose while Rick was compressing the Mini's chest. Tuffy was dead.

What could cause a Mini to die so quickly without showing any of the normal colic signs? He had not pawed or sweated. He had not gotten up and down. In retrospect Rosie thought he might have had trouble seeing the night before, but his Sunday morning signs were reportedly just a rapid, progressive depression to death.

Everyone suspected a plant toxicity, and we searched the arena fence line twice. We found just a little crab grass in the arena—no nightshade, yews, cherry trees, or other suspicious plants along the fence. I checked the tube of Bute paste. There were still 7 grams in the 12-gram tube. Tuffy had indeed received just 1 gram per day for five days, including the first gram I gave him on Wednesday. He was short, but fat—about 400 pounds. I strongly suspected the Bute had caused a perforating ulcer and the Mini died of peritonitis shock. While everyone wanted to know why he died, no one wanted to blame anyone. Everyone was very emotional, and Tuffy was buried within a half hour, without an autopsy. I count his death as a probable Bute hypersensitivity toxicity, which I had previously seen possibly nine times in 33 years. These three cases of acute, severe Grade IV laminitis are very similar to the case of Sandy McDaniel, a similarly obese Paint mare reported here.

Tuffy's death, in hindsight, was almost surely toxic shock from a perforated ulcer, caused by the Bute (24). I should have reminded Rosie when she called on Thursday to report that Tuffy was "much better," that she could give just 1/2 gram or even skip a day. The minimum effective dose is in the eye of the person watching the horse day to day. That can be different for two different observers.

All the Bute toxicity ulcer studies were done with healthy ponies. To explain the difference between the large and prolonged doses that I often had to use to save horses with laminitis, I have come to belief that Bute first goes to the sight of the active inflammation, then excess Bute attacks the intestinal lining, causing ulcers. Just 1 gram of Bute is an overdose to a normal pony with no inflammation.

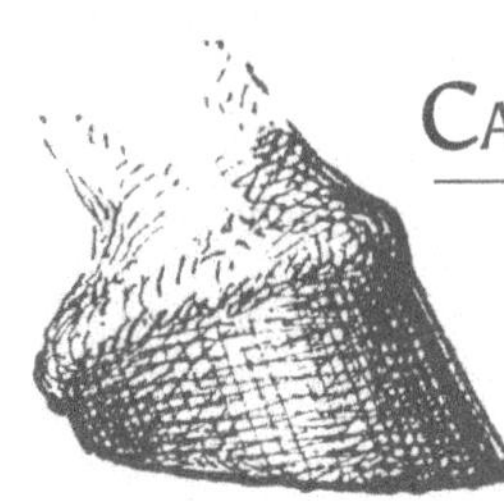

## Case Study

# "King"

### *Saved Because of Three Different Sets of Eyes*

KING, A 15-YEAR-OLD CLYDESDALE GELDING, was owned and cared for by Jean Adams, a very experienced and capable horsewoman. She had excellent judgement about what she could do herself, and when she needed to call the vet. When Jean called me on July 9, 2002, she was concerned King might have a mild case of laminitis. King had been "slightly off" while roaming his paddock "for four or five days." As usual, I was behind schedule that day, but I would always try to see any suspected acute laminitis case the same day the owner called because untreated laminitis can progress very quickly.

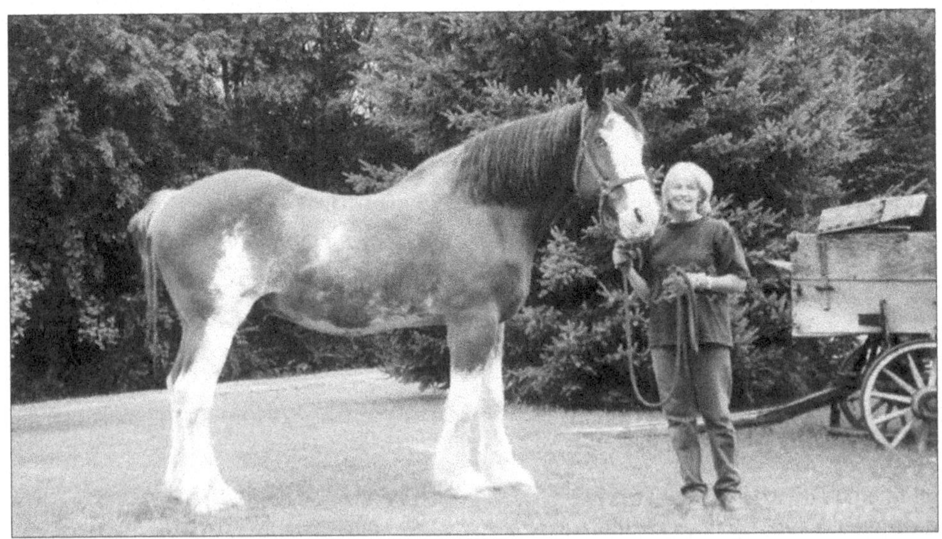

*King*

King was a very stoic horse, and he showed no tenderness at all where an abscess had opened at the bulb of the heel. He totally ignored my pounding on his front hoof walls with a hoof tester, which would elicit an immediate reaction from a normal horse with acute laminitis. King was not at all overweight, and he was kept with three other horses in a grassless paddock with unrestricted grass hay. I could not find a digital pulse. When Jean trotted King away from me on a lead line, he was certainly rougher than the light horses I'm used to looking at. After watching him trot several times, I could not say he was lame. Jean knew him much better and still felt he was "off."

While I was admittedly rushed, I told Jean that King did not have laminitis. I left no treatment, but I asked Jean to call me back if he got worse. As I was driving home, it occurred to me that King's paddock is heavily wooded on two sides. I called Jean and asked her to walk those two fence lines looking for any weeds King might have eaten over the fence. I asked her to especially look for nightshade, which I have seen cause laminitis eight or ten times.

Jean called back two days later saying that King was a little worse. Now it was easy for me to see his head bob about half the time, when trotting on the lead line. He was also noticeably sore turning around to come back. I could still find no digital pulse through King's heavily feathered and thick-skinned fetlocks, and he still showed no reaction to my hoof testers.

I decided to use a variation of a flexion test which I had stumbled upon 20 years earlier. King readily picked up either front foot for me, so I held up his right front leg for 60 seconds. When asked to trot off after standing on his left front leg for 60 seconds, King was obviously more lame then when we had watched him trot minutes earlier. Next, I held up his left front leg for 60 seconds, and when he trotted off his lameness switched to head bobbing on his right front for the first 5 or 6 strides, then went back to his left front.

I treated King with 12 cc Bute IV, and I asked Jean to give the nearly 2,000-pound King just 2 grams of Bute paste per day the next 6 days. This was a very mild dose for a draft horse, but he was not at all fat and it was a very mild case. Jean asked if diapering his feet would help. Diapers and duct tape will cushion the feet and prevent dried mud from packing in the feet, putting pressure on the soles of horses with laminitis. Jean did this, a difficult job for a small lady with King's huge feet, and I'm sure it helped him walk his paddock more easily. I never confine a horse with acute laminitis to a stall. They need to walk for optimum circulation to heal the laminae.

Before I left, Jean and I walked the two wooded sides of his fence line together, since there was nothing Jean was feeding him that could have caused his laminitis. I only found one small nightshade plant about three feet out of reach of any of the horses, with nothing eaten from it. We did find a number of other weeds that were obviously eaten, but only one seemed suspicious to me. Its leaves were similar to the nightshade I was used to seeing.

The University of Illinois has an extension office about two miles from Jean's farm, so I took in a sample of the suspicious plant. The nice folks identified my plant as an Elderberry bush, with no likely toxicity. One of the ladies, Margie Bjorkman, was a horse owner. Margie asked if she could come check the fence lines herself. As Margie walked the fence lines with Jean and I, it didn't take her five minutes to spot a wild cherry tree in the thick woods. One of the branches reached over the fence and the Clydesdale had eaten it like a giraffe, nine to ten feet off the ground! Wild cherry trees can be difficult for a novice to identify, but they are a well-known cause of laminitis.

Twenty years earlier, in a very similar situation, I had let myself be overruled by more experienced veterinarians on second opinion who de-nerved the horse for chronic navicular disease (*see Peter's story*). It wasn't until a month later when we put the horse to sleep, because his coffin bones dropped through his soles without further warning, that we discovered he had been grazing from oak trees overhanging his sandy round pen. Thank goodness I learned from my mistake.

A week later, after King was off the very low dose Bute for a day, he was moving much better, and he passed the trotting test just fine. While fat horses take six to eight weeks to recover from acute laminitis, thin or fit horses can be fully recovered in three to ten days.

# ~SECTION VIII~

## Owner Treated Cases

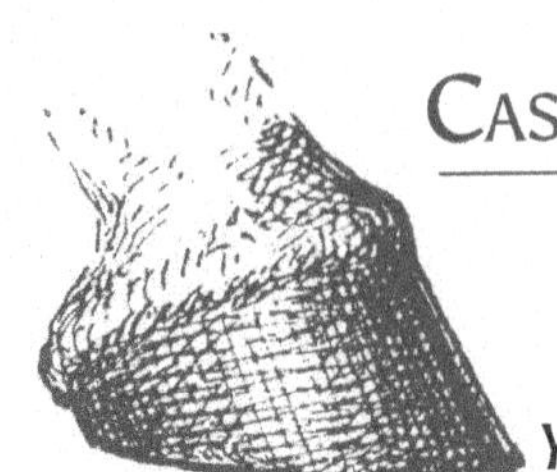

## Case Study

# "Tequila"

*Young Paint Gelding Saved by Owner/Advocate*

**WHEN LUCY HEARD I WAS** publishing a book of laminitis cases, she immediately asked if Tequila's story was in the book. I had remembered that Tequila, a currently 15-year-old Paint gelding, had a laminitis attack about ten years earlier. I did not remember any special circumstances to include in this book. Lucy could not have disagreed more. "You saved his life!" she insisted. While I saw about 30 laminitis cases most years, Tequila's case was the scariest case of laminitis Lucy had ever seen, and she remembered it clearly. She reminded me that Tequila had not been able to move at all before I saw him. I reviewed his records and decided to write up one more case, because Lucy saved his life, not me.

For the past 20 years, Lucy has kept six to eight horses in her very nice backyard farm and stable with barn, paddocks, and small pastures. One or two of the horses were usually owned and ridden by Lucy and her husband, but the rest were retired geldings, whose owners from the city only occasionally visited their horses. Lucy's skilled husband built the excellent barn and fencing, and Lucy did nearly all the daily chores by herself. Lucy had taken my Horse Health Care classes at the local junior college in 1995 when she started her horse boarding operation. However, I had never been her vet, until she called me to see Tequila on May 2, 2005.

Tequila was about 150 pounds overweight and had Grade II acute laminitis when I saw him. He was obese from very good alfalfa hay, and one hour a day of lush spring pasture. Tequila reportedly had been unable to move three days earlier, when Lucy's regular vet told her, "He's foundered, put him in the stall and get shoes on him right away." He gave him a shot of Banamine, and Lucy followed up with 3 grams of Bute paste twice a day the next two days before calling me. She remembered from my Horse Health Care class ten years earlier, that I did not advise shoes or stall confinement for laminitis. Tequila had received 12 grams of Bute while locked in his stall the 48 hours immediately prior to my first visit.

Tequila also had an abscess in his left front hoof, treated four weeks earlier, which I had to reopen and drain. We then applied iodine and Epsom salts and wrapped his left front foot with a diaper and duct tape. I showed Lucy how to shake the alfalfa leaves out of Tequila's hay and feed him the stems from just two flakes of hay three times a day. I asked her to leave Tequila in her 40-foot indoor sand round pen 24/7. His feet had been trimmed fairly short the week earlier, so there was no extra toe or heel for me to remove. Because of his extra 150 pounds I wanted the sand to distribute his weight over the entire sole rather than just the wall with a horseshoe.

I rechecked Tequila three days later. I had to drill out the abscess this time, replace the diaper and duct tape over iodine and Epsom salts, and emphasize to Lucy the importance of keeping the abscess hole clean. The laminitis was being controlled quite well with just 1 gram of Bute twice a day, sand footing, and the hay stems with few leaves.

A week later, Tequila was more lame again, and I found mud packed in the abscess hole. Lucy soon became quite proficient using the diapers and did not need to call me again for a month. By then Tequila's feet were grown out, he had lost close to 100 pounds, and he was actually tapered off Bute more quickly than I expected. Usually, it takes about six weeks for all the endotoxins to be cleared from a horse as fat as Tequila, but he had cleared it within a month, perhaps because he was younger and more active than most foundered horses. X-rays on my final visit showed minimal damage, and to Lucy's credit, Tequila has never had a relapse in over ten

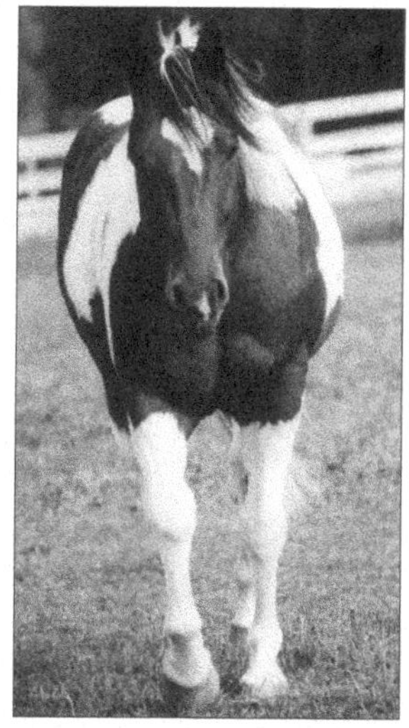

*Tequila*

years. He is still a very easy keeper, but Lucy has never allowed him to get fat again. He wears a muzzle anytime the pasture is growing fast, and he holds his weight very well with minimal alfalfa or grain.

I had only seen Tequila four times, and he responded and was fully cured much quicker than I expected, despite the complicating abscess and extra weight. Obviously, Lucy had done her work every day with him. That is probably why it was not such a significant case to me as it was to her. She is the one who saved his life, by calling for a second opinion on day three when he was standing in his stall on massive doses of Bute. His month with laminitis has not once been an issue since 2005.

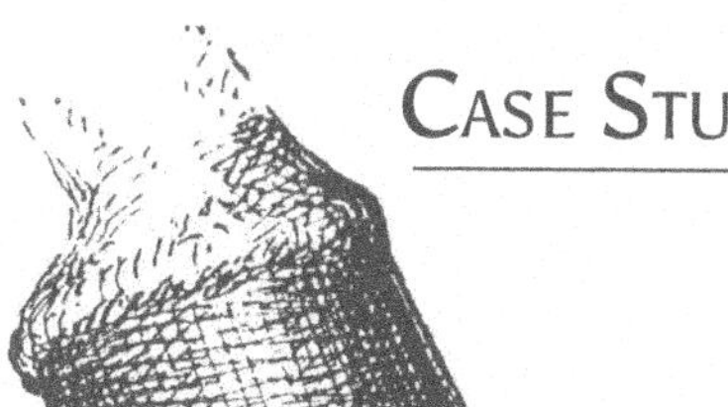

## Case Study

# "911"

### *Repeat Feed Room Raider*

911 WAS A LARGE FOX hunting gelding, owned, cared for, and ridden by a doctor. 911 was a very easy keeper, a very pleasant and friendly horse to work with, and a very good mix of 3/4 Thoroughbred, and probably 1/4 Percheron. He simply had a very agreeable personality, and it was always a pleasure to work with him.

On a Memorial Day weekend in the 1990s, the owners were out of town, and one of the doctor's nurses was left in charge of the horses. Sally called me early Saturday morning to report that 911 had gotten out of his stall overnight, knocked the lid off the grain barrel, and eaten probably 30 to 40 pounds of sweet feed.

Sally felt so badly about apparently having forgotten to latch 911's stall door the night before that she wanted to pay for my trip, the gallon of mineral oil, and shots of Bute and Dipyrone I gave 911 to prevent laminitis and colic. I assured her that was not necessary, but the greatest danger was the possibility of laminitis showing up about 48 hours after such a grain binge. Hopefully, the oil would speed the passage of the grain overload and prevent the absorption of endotoxins in the gut that can trigger laminitis in the feet. If some endotoxins did escape the gut, the single 2-gram dose of Bute was intended to prevent inflammation of the laminae.

I also asked Sally to withhold all grain, alfalfa, and especially the lush spring pasture until the danger of laminitis from the grain over-load had passed. This was before grazing muzzles became popular, but 911 was definitely the type of horse to eventually benefit from one. The week went fine with no hint of soreness.

The episode was repeated a couple of months later when 911's owners were home. While I administered the Bute, Dipyrone (to relax his intestine), and mineral oil via stomach tube, the doctor felt she was the dummy who forgot to check the stall latch. Once again 911 showed no hint of laminitis the week following his grain binge and our laminitis prevention treatment. Later, the owners saw 911 occasionally play with his stall latch over the top of his door. On October 29th that same year, he got into the sweet feed again and they realized that he had learned to open the latch with his lips and chin. They no longer felt guilty, but did not call me that morning since 911 had not gotten colic or laminitis from his two previous incidents.

Two days later, 911 was very foot-sore. He had an easily detectable digital pulse and was sore to the hoof testers at both front toes. He hurt much worse turning either direction than walking straight away. I gave him 10 cc (2 grams) of Bute IV and left 30 cc with the doctor for her to give, as needed, at the minimum effective dose. He had been hunting barefoot, so there was no need to remove shoes from his very tough black feet. I simply rasped off a square toe to ease breakover and rasped down his heels a little to get better frog pressure. I then asked for him to be kept in a smaller dirt lot, with no pasture, no box stall at night, and no grain until he was totally sound.

I was called back on November 15th because of lingering mild soreness two weeks after my only treatment visit. X-rays that day showed zero rotation or sinking of the coffin bone. The doctor had given the 30 cc of Bute in decreasing doses the first week of November and 911 seemed to quickly respond, but after two weeks he still was not 100% sound. His digital pulse was barely detectable. I did not give any more medications. I simply touched up his squared toes and lowered heels with my rasp and asked for a little longer time in the dry lot and no stall time at night. The lingering soreness was gone by the end of the week, and 911 had a great fox hunt on Thanksgiving Day.

Leaner horses can fully recover in less time. I believe the endotoxins absorbed into the blood, in addition to causing inflammation in the laminae, can be stored in fat cells. At the extremes, a really fat horse can take six or eight weeks to recover from a really severe case of acute laminitis that a really lean horse could be fully recovered from in six to eight days. The recovery time is directly related to the length of time after the acute laminitis starts before proper treatment is started. If commonly prescribed treatments such as vasodilators, stall confinement, and "therapeutic" shoes are used, too many never recover.

Over 42 years, I have had at least 100 horses get into the feed room in the middle of the night. If the owners called the next morning, not one of them ever got laminitis after receiving my standard gallon of mineral oil and 10 cc injections of Bute and Dipyrone. Some of those who did not receive my treatment (like 911, Caesar, Surprise once, and Charlie) had to be treated for laminitis two or three days later. Prophylactic intervention is always better than treatment of progressive symptoms after the disease becomes evident.

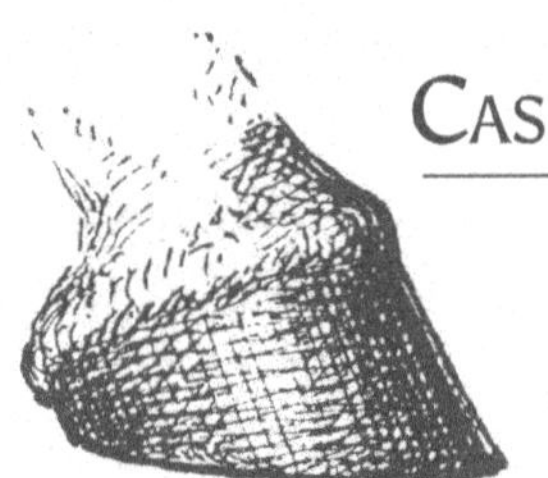

Case Study

# "Bill"

## *Special Patient for Over 30 Years*

BILL WAS A VERY SPECIAL patient for over 30 years. He was just four years younger than my wife's Surprise, and their careers had many similarities. They lived just a few miles apart, and they attended many of the same events, shows, fox hunts and trail rides for about 20 of those years. I did Bill's pre-purchase exam for Megan in 1982, when he was a barely broke 2-year-old Paint gelding. He immediately impressed me as a very confident, sound, and friendly horse. Megan participated in dressage and jumping, and while Bill's primarily Quarter Horse conformation was not ideal, Bill was willing to learn anything Megan wanted to teach him over the years. He fox hunted when he was just a four year old, started eventing soon after that, and saw some success in both the dressage and hunter show rings despite his loud color and stout conformation. A couple times, when I needed a client's horse for myself, or an out-of-town visitor, I borrowed Bill for the day. Whenever I rode Bill, I always felt like he had "a leg at each corner." He was one of my all-time favorite patients because of his personality and versatility.

When Bill was 19, he no longer could hold up to the level, frequency, and intensity of riding and lessons that Megan still enjoyed. I arranged for another client with two young girls to buy Bill for a dollar. He taught them both how to ride, and they and their mom continued to take Bill on occasional short trail rides into his early 30s. At both of his homes Bill was personally cared for morning and night by his riders, and he always shared both of his five-acre pastures with one or two other horses who came and went over the years. He was very rarely in a stall day or night.

Throughout the 30 consecutive years I was Bill's vet, I remember he had just a couple very mild colics, which were cured within an hour or two. His occasional mild soreness was usually due to too much jumping or dressage for a horse with his conformation and cured with a week off.

Checking Bill's digital pulse showed rest was usually all he needed. However, he did have at least three or four bouts of mild acute laminitis over the years. It was usually after eating fast-growing spring grass. For each bout of acute laminitis, Bill was treated with Bute for just two or three days at most. Bill was always very active, and never fat, so simple adjustment in pasture time was all he ever needed.

Bill never had ideal tough, round feet, but his owners always took very good care of the feet God gave him. He was shod most of the year when he was younger, but he was barefoot most winters, and most of the second half of his life. Because Bill was predisposed to laminitis, I have no doubt that if he had not been seen every day by his observant and educated owners, he would have been the type of horse who one day showed up foundered due to what they now call "subclinical laminitis." To me "sub-acute laminitis" is really just unnoticed, undiagnosed, or too often misdiagnosed, mild acute laminitis. If all horses received the care Bill had his whole life, most horses would live useful lives well into their 30s. And far fewer horses would founder.

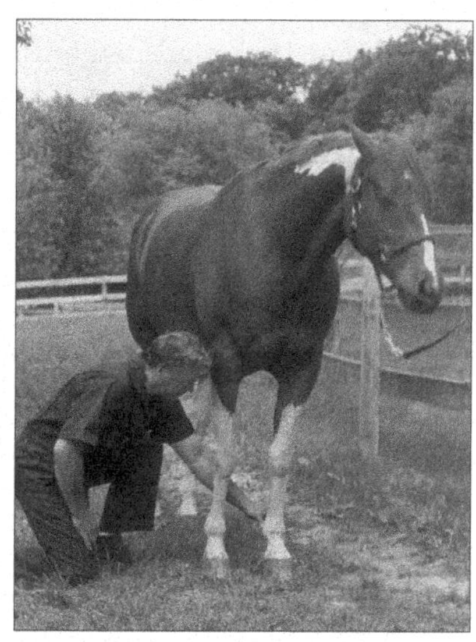

*Bill with Dr. Frederick*

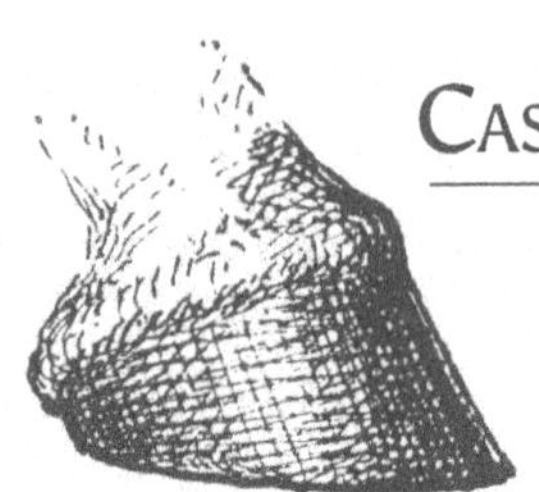

## Case Study

# "Bobby"

*Bad Advice from a Nosy Neighbor*

BOBBY WAS A HOMEBRED AQHA gelding. I was his vet from age 15 until I had to put him to sleep at just 25. With his super long hair and very poor muscling, Bobby very obviously had early-onset Cushing's disease when I first met him at 15. He needed to be body clipped once or twice every summer. However, this was 1995, before pergolide was widely prescribed and well before all the low starch grains were available in the feed stores.

Bobby's first laminitis attack was not until age 22, in June when his pasture was growing very fast. He recovered 100% with just two to three weeks of decreasing doses of Bute, no pasture, and just two vet visits. Mary was especially careful and worried because she told me Bobby's mother had died from laminitis when Bobby was a yearling.

Bobby had two more very mild attacks the next year, which were successfully treated even quicker than his first one. The following year, at age 24, Bobby had just one attack, again treated successfully in just a week. Bobby was never fat and keeping weight on him without setting off laminitis was becoming a problem. Mary had a large truckload of sand dumped in his small paddock by the barn to provide softer footing when he was not allowed on pasture. About this time Mary was getting a lot of advice from her neighbor, a former client of mine who had her own ideas about everything, and no interest in anything I said. She would feed and care for Bobby whenever Mary was out of town. At age 25, Mary followed the neighbor's severely limited feeding restrictions, and Bobby was a rack of bones. I had to put him to sleep that summer with uncontrollable "thumps," an uncontrolled fluttering of the equine diaphragm, usually associated with dehydration and low calcium. It was probably triggered by malnutrition from all the things the neighbor convinced Mary not to feed Bobby.

Without the neighbor's daily conflicting advice, I believe Bobby would have lived very comfortably, and mostly drug free, for another five years at least.

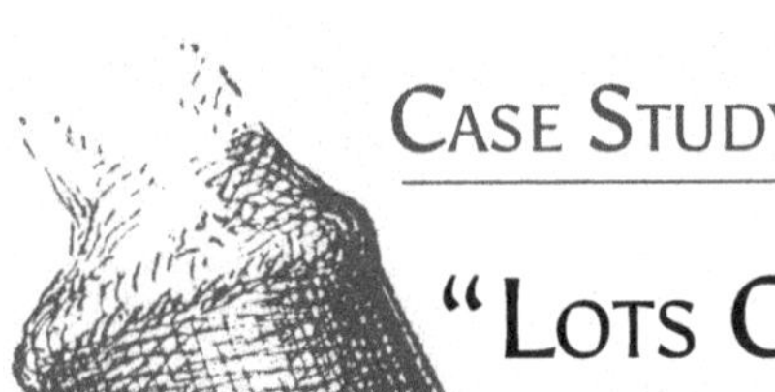

Case Study

# "Lots O' Dots" and "Spirit"

## *Two Very Simple and Quickly Resolved Grade IV Cases*

LOTS O' DOTS AND SPIRIT are two horses who illustrate how simply and quickly even severe acute laminitis can be cured, if treated promptly and correctly. Both horses had been patients of mine for a number of years, and had very responsible, intelligent, and attentive owners when they were found very sore in their stalls at evening feedings.

Lots O' Dots was a horse who had never had a significant lameness of any kind prior to his attack of severe Grade IV acute laminitis. Dots had a long career as a lead pony and was about 20 when Cindy bought the Appaloosa gelding at Arlington Park to use as a lesson horse in her new stable. That was 1994, and over the next 12 years, Cindy said at least 50 different riders of all ages learned to canter for the first time on Dots. Cindy's favorite story described when a green rider slipped off Dots in a schooling show and Dots continued jumping the beginner course without her!

When Dots refused to come to his feed bucket for dinner on Friday night, April 1, 1998, Cindy was immediately called to his stall. Cindy found Dots had a mild fever of 100.7 degrees, but he resisted moving around in his stall. Despite his fabulous manners under saddle, Dots was always a suspicious horse in the stall, and he normally had a hard time standing still whenever a vet or a thermometer was around.

I was out to dinner when Cindy called. I had known Cindy and the horse well for years, and I trusted her description of Dots' problem. Dots had never been overweight, but Cindy was describing classic acute laminitis. He had finished his morning feed, but it had been raining all day, so he had not been turned out. Since he had no lessons scheduled, he stayed in his stall. And now he strongly resisted letting Cindy pick up either front foot. He was not shod, but he had properly trimmed natural feet. On my request, she was able to force him out of his stall and get him to walk a little in the aisle. He improved some, but she reported he obviously hurt worse turning in the aisle to return to his stall. I also asked Cindy to check for a pulse at the base of Dots' sesamoid bones, which she found easily. I prescribed emergency treatment over the phone because I trusted Cindy's description completely. This was one of the very few times in 42 years I deferred a visit to confirm a severe acute laminitis diagnosis. Dots was barefoot, and I asked Cindy to give him just 2 grams of Bute paste, hose his feet with cold water in the wash rack, then turn him loose in her lighted indoor sand arena overnight with three flakes of grass hay in different areas. I felt this would encourage him to walk from flake to flake most of the night.

When I checked on Dots the following morning, he showed no sign of his laminitis to hoof testers or turning in the aisle, or even a palpable digital pulse. With Dots loose in the arena, I clapped my hands and he bolted off, just as I would expect this always alert horse to do on any other day. The most likely cause of Dots' laminitis was very good mixed hay that had significantly more alfalfa than usual for this barn, combined with his abnormally long stall confinement. If he had been turned out that morning, the laminitis likely wouldn't have been noticed until the next morning.

Sadly, Dots was euthanized in 2007, in his mid-30s, due to recurring penile cancer, but he never had another attack of laminitis, and his hooves never showed any sign of his one-day attack of severe Grade IV acute laminitis.

Six and a half years after Dots, on August 28, 2004, a Saturday evening, Marie called to tell me Spirit, her 10-year-old black American Saddlebred mare seemed off when she went to the barn for evening feeding. When Marie, a full-time hospital nurse, and the primary caretaker of her family's five horses, tried to bring Spirit out of her stall to see what was wrong, she found the mare very lame all around and called me on my cell phone while she stood beside her immobile horse. Marie had never seen acute laminitis before, but her calm and reliable observations and answers to my questions made the diagnosis very clear. She easily found the throbbing pulse behind the fetlock. It is very dangerous to make a habit of treating horses over the phone, but, like Cindy and Dots, I was very familiar with Marie, Spirit, and her barn.

I asked Marie to give Spirit 3 grams of the Bute tablets she had left over from an older horse's earlier treatment, to hose the mare's feet for 15 minutes, and to turn her loose overnight in her sand indoor arena. I asked her to put small piles of hay stems in several spots after she shook most of the alfalfa leaves out in the aisle. I must emphasize that feeding hay in the sand is a short-term practice, and I never recommend feeding leafy hays or grain in sand arenas. Grass hay or well-shaken leafy hay for a few days has never caused a problem for my patients. But horses are very likely to eat too much sand going after loose leaves and spilled grain in an arena with the associated risk of sand colic. Like Dots, Spirit was barefoot, so there was no need to remove any shoes.

Marie called after church Sunday morning to report that Spirit was moving much better and that her digital pulse was dramatically softer, but she was still sore when brought out of the arena and walked on the concrete aisle. She assured me I did not need to make a Sunday call, but agreed to give 2 grams of Bute tablets, hose the mare's feet again, and leave Spirit in the sand arena with just hay stems and water.

Monday morning, Marie reported her patient to be 90% back to normal, even walking on the concrete. Her pulse was hard to find, even for the nurse. We agreed to one more gram of Bute, and she left Spirit in the arena two more days and nights, until Marie was convinced that the horse was absolutely sound Wednesday morning—48 hours after her last dose of Bute, and after four days and nights in the sand arena.

I was able to identify the cause of Spirit's laminitis by asking Marie questions. The alfalfa hay field next to the pasture was in bloom. It was too short for a second cutting, but Marie had been stopping by the alfalfa field each morning and evening to give each horse a treat on the way in and out of the barn. Because Spirit was the leanest of her horses, Marie would let the Saddlebred graze the alfalfa field longer than the other four horses. Marie had left the horses in their stalls that rainy Saturday and given them extra alfalfa hay for the day. Too much rich alfalfa, and too little exercise triggered the laminitis event.

After more than four decades of practicing veterinary medicine, I still believe the second rule of good medicine is that you must examine the patient (the first rule is "do no harm"). There can be a rare exception to the second rule when you have trusted and qualified help. These two cases are two more examples of why I have never believed that laminitis is a "mysterious disease" that will require millions more dollars of research before veterinarians can hope to someday understand the disease frequently reported as "incurable and often fatal."

Restoring optimum circulation by reducing inflammation and edema, the minimum effective daily dose of Bute (as long as necessary), often cold water, sometimes Lasix, always identifying and eliminating the cause(s), and providing a soft place to walk on properly trimmed and frequent-cleaned feet always works, when laminitis is caught in the acute stage. Extended stall rest, venograms, vasodilators, anticoagulants, anti-endotoxin serum, special shoes and pads, tendon severing surgery, "hoof realignments," etc., do not always save acute laminitis cases, even in the most prestigious hospitals, with the smartest veterinarians, and the most skillful farriers.

Every case of chronic laminitis is preceded by acute laminitis. Severe acute laminitis is much easier to recognize than mild acute laminitis. But the severe cases have a much shorter window of opportunity to institute correct treatment than the slower mild cases. Both Spirit and Dots would likely have required longer treatment (and been much more likely to have suffered some laminar damage) if they had been forced to wait for the vet until Monday morning, in their stalls and on regular feed, before starting treatment.

In my 42 years in the same practice, it has invariably been the mild cases which were much more likely to suffer some rotation than the severe cases. Owners call much more quickly, and listen much better, when their horses are in serious pain from severe acute laminitis. The severe acute cases are normally seen as quickly as severe colics. With mild acute laminitis in pasture horses there can be rotation before the owner even notices the horse is lame, although it usually takes weeks. Also, with milder laminitis, owners sometimes resist feeding, stabling, and shoeing recommendations. Owners often think they are feeding a mixed hay with very little alfalfa. Shaking the hay out on a concrete aisle, then picking up the stems frequently leaves a very impressive pile of alfalfa leaves. Unfortunately, sometimes the horse has to get worse before some owners or trainers really start to listen and understand the seriousness of the condition.

A note on stall confinement: Confinement in a stall causes the blood to stagnate in the feet. A walk refreshes the feet with fresh blood, and the horse walks much better. But if the horse is then put back in the stall the inadequate circulation to the laminae returns. Just as stall confinement increases the risk of colic, it makes acute laminitis treatment much more difficult. A horse's feet were designed to expand and contract. Stalls and shoes inhibit the optimum circulation so necessary for full healing.

This stall confinement problem is mostly ignored by hospital veterinarians, but a January 1984 laminitis case, which I have included in this book (*see M.J.*), removed any doubt I might have ever had about the detrimental effects of stall confinement on laminar circulation. A well-fed, 7-year-old Arab gelding developed acute Grade II laminitis due to a combination of grain, alfalfa, a week of oral dexamethazone (5 mg/day), and excessive stall confinement. We stopped the grain and dexamethazone and tried to shake the alfalfa out of the hay, but while the laminitis was relatively mild, it proved to be a persistent case. At first 2 grams of Bute paste per day made him walk fine, but if we skipped the Bute for a day, the short stride was back.

This was a backyard horse owned by a busy and successful businesswoman. She did not really believe her horse was "foundered," and he wasn't yet. She resisted the feeding restrictions, and only partly complied with the turnout requests, because "it was cold" in Chicago in January. Overnight turnout was out of the question for this owner. What saved the horse from foundering that winter was that she insisted that I come every day to personally administer the Bute paste, the only time this has happened in 42 years.

The silver lining in this annoying case was that I learned something as I checked the horse's progress every day. The laminitis took about three weeks to fully resolve, and I learned that each morning I could easily feel a stronger-than-normal digital pulse, but if I took the horse out and walked him in the snow for just two or three minutes, the palpable pulse would disappear. When the horse returned to the stall, within five minutes I could feel his digital pulse again.

I have believed since I started vet school in 1970 that the strength of the digital pulse is directly related to the degree of inflammation within the hoof. I intuitively believed the body had a homeostatic oxygen sensing mechanism, something I would not find in the literature until 2006 (27). The body senses insufficient oxygen, and sympathetic nerves constrict other arteries, redirecting more blood under higher pressure to the hypoxic laminae. Dr. Chris Pollitt's classic circulatory casts (7) showed this in 1990, but he has never believed my interpretation of his excellent research. The minimum effective daily dose of Bute is not so much for pain control, but to reduce inflammation which allows more normal circulation to the laminae, which is trapped between the hoof and the coffin bone.

Finally, horses must walk for optimum circulation in their feet. Stall confinement makes their feet "stock up," just the same as their legs stock up when they don't get enough exercise. Human medicine realized 25 years ago that patients heal better when they get them out of bed and make them move. It's past time for veterinary medicine to come to the same conclusion.

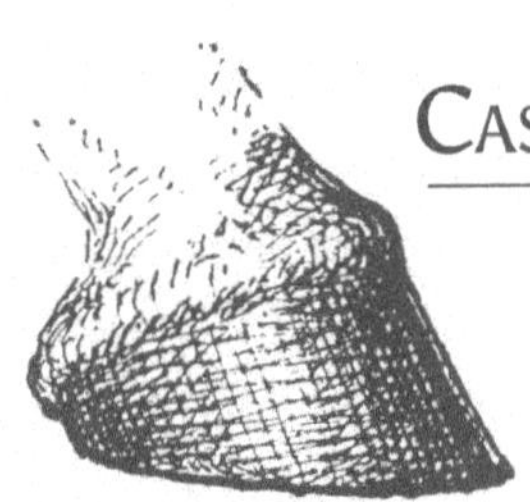

# Case Study

## "Maverick"

### *5 Years of Well-Controlled Laminitis*

MAVERICK WAS A 19-YEAR-OLD Tennessee Walker gelding with the same slow, easy keeper metabolism as the other horses in this group. I cared for him since he was purchased as a 4-year-old. He had his first mild laminitis attack at age 5. He was in a very lush 60-acre hillside pasture 24/7. The horses get very fat in this particular field every summer, which is just too hilly to be an excellent hayfield. Most of the horses just got fat without getting laminitis, because they began grazing before it grew so high. Although the lack of sudden changes seems to reduce the incidence of laminitis, I believe horses allowed to graze fields like this are more likely to eventually develop this disease.

Maverick's first acute laminitis, at age 5, was identified very early and successfully treated simply, by taking him off the field and putting him on gradually lower doses of Bute for a couple weeks. His farrier was very upset that I did not prescribe therapeutic shoes and more restrictions, but Maverick was quickly back to normal after just squaring the toe and lowering his heels. There was no separation of the white line, dropping of the sole, or any other hoof changes.

Two years later Maverick had another attack that was treated just as simply and successfully, again with no visible hoof damage. Maverick was born with very well shaped and tough hooves that withstood periodic laminitis episodes if treated promptly.

At the age of 10, Maverick was moved to a new smaller field. The four acres of grass for three horses never grew more than six inches tall but Maverick started having more frequent flare-ups on the smaller and shorter pasture. The owners, who did not live on the farm now, had primary responsibility to recognize the flare-ups and initiate treatment. Since Maverick was out walking around 24/7, I'm sure there were multiple minor flare-ups they did not recognize. Maverick had a couple abscesses over the next nine years, and he did start developing separation of his white line.

Most horses will show abscess pain by refusing to put weight on that leg, but Maverick would walk swinging his front foot in a big arc away from his body. Normally such an odd walk would make the vet look inside his elbow for the source of the pain, but both times I found a typical abscess in the now separated white line.

Maverick now needs to wear a muzzle most of the pasture season, from about April 15 to September 15, depending on pasture growth. Often, we get a summer drought in this area in July or August with dormant pastures, but rapid growing lush pasture returns if the rains come back for a week or more. Warm rainy weather often gives me a laminitis cluster of three or more cases to treat within a week, whether it is May/June or August/September.

Maverick's owners know what to watch for and usually would just come over to buy a tube of Bute paste when they need it. Otherwise, Maverick still goes on long trail rides almost anytime they want.

# ~SECTION IX~

## Recurring Cases

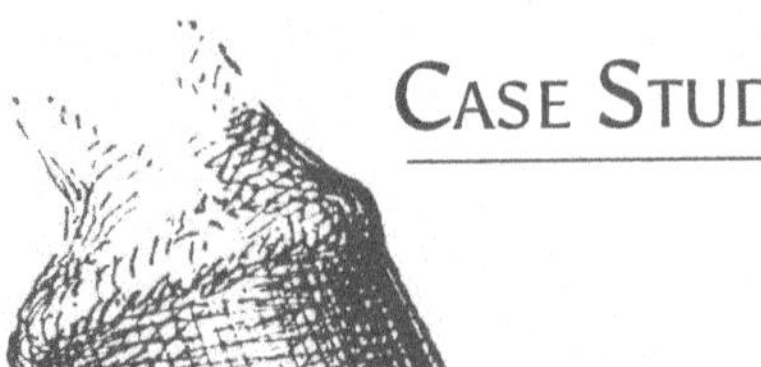

## Case Study

# "M.J."

### *My First Example that Stall Confinement Raises Digital Pulse*

M.J. WAS A DELIGHTFUL 26-YEAR-OLD black Arabian gelding whom I knew since he was purchased as a 3-year-old in 1980. After a short stint with a professional trainer, he was then an excellent backyard family horse.

M.J.'s first health problem was a swollen sheath as a 7-year-old in January of 1984. I cleaned his greasy sheath, and I gave his owners a combination antibiotic and dexamethazone powder to be given orally in divided doses over the next week, while his sheath was cleaned every other day.

By the end of the week, M.J. had his first of what would be many bouts of laminitis. M.J.'s owner initially noted just "stiffness in his shoulders," but I observed bilateral sore front feet, sensitivity to hoof testers at both front toes, and an increased digital pulse pressure in both front feet. The dexamethazone, not more than 5 mg per day, may have contributed to M.J.'s first acute laminitis attack more or less than his very good alfalfa hay, his grain, his cresty neck, his reduced winter exercise, or his being stall-bound on rubber mats when his owner felt it was too cold for him to be outside.

We immediately stopped the dexamethazone, grain, and alfalfa hay, but I was unable to convince the owner that his feet would heal faster if he were allowed to wander in his paddock.

Nevertheless, he needed 2 grams of Bute on a daily basis, and while we were able to drop to 1 gram of Bute paste per day by the end of the week, he would be sore again if we skipped a day. His mild case of laminitis proved to be very persistent, mostly due to the owner's insistence on keeping him in his stall during the January cold weather.

The owner was a successful business executive, but marginal horse caretaker. She insisted that I personally visit to administer his Bute paste every day. While I considered this an unnecessary inconvenience, it gave me the opportunity to check his digital pulse each morning while he was recovering.

What I learned in January of 1984 was that each morning for nearly six weeks, M.J. would have an easily detectable increased digital pulse pressure in both front feet, but not in his hind feet. Before administering his daily gram of Bute paste, if I would take him out and walk him in the snow for just two or three minutes, his digital pulse pressure would disappear. After standing in his stall for ten minutes, the pulse pressure would again be easily detectable.

Ten years later, Dr. Chris Pollitt released an excellent video tape (9) of his hoof circulation studies, which clearly showed that the alternating compression and relaxation of a normal, flexible, unshod hoof, during the alternating phases of a horse's stride significantly assists the circulation within the hoof. A stall-bound horse, particularly shod or on rubber mats, loses the circulatory benefit of alternating pressures on the hoof.

After about six weeks, M.J. was off the Bute and absolutely sound. That summer, his farrier could find no evidence of any white line separation or sole dropping. Unfortunately, over the next ten years with chronic over feeding and inadequate exercise, M.J. suffered four more bouts of laminitis. Each time he would fully recover in two to six weeks and be absolutely sound with normal hooves and no continued medication.

In August of 1994, a two-week bout of his laminitis was linked to deadly nightshade, which he had eaten through the fence of his heavily wooded paddock. Once again, he recovered nicely.

However, about this time M.J. developed serious heaves from his 15 years of confinement in a rather tight barn. For the next two years he was heavily medicated with daily antihistamines. I was hesitant to use any dexamethazone because of his original laminitis episode, and I was still unsuccessful in convincing his owner that he would be better off outside away from the humid, musty barn. She began sending her husband to feed him, because she didn't like seeing him experiencing respiratory distress.

Two and a half years later, in April 1997, likely after a couple unrecognized and untreated laminitis bouts, he had substantial separation at the white line and dropped soles. I was finally able to convince the owner that M.J. would be an excellent kids' first horse for a client of mine out in the country. After moving to the country, M.J. did not spend one night locked in a stall, breathing fine with no antihistamines. Unfortunately, on much better pasture the first three years he had serious flare-ups each spring when warm weather and rains made the grass especially rich. In 1999 an ambitious farrier gave him modified hoof resections (the only time ever in my practice) and put him in heart bar shoes for 18 months. He was barefoot after the fall of 2000, and had only one laminitis flare up the following three years after grazing shrubbery on the other side of his fence. Three young boys had a blast learning to ride him during those three years.

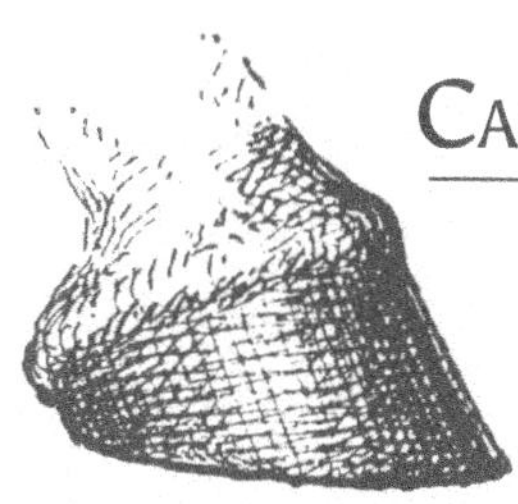

## Case Study

# "Paso Rojo"

### *A Poor Veterinarian-Client Relationship*

THE FIRST TIME I MET Rojo and Bonnie was for a second opinion "pre-purchase exam"—for a free horse. Bonnie wanted to know if Rojo could be saved, as his owner's only other alternative was to put him to sleep. Bonnie had some prior experience with horses and thought she could save him. The owner also wanted to give him a chance, but she had a very specific list of feed and medication requirements for Rojo's chronic laminitis. Otherwise, she was ready to put him down at the age of 10! The pergolide at the time was to be about $2.50 per day for the rest of his life. The designer feeds were almost double the cost of conventional grains, and there were a couple expensive supplements that the "seller" also insisted he must have every day.

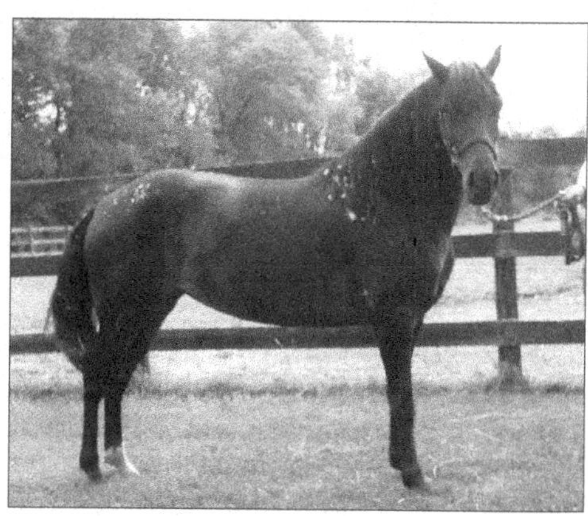

*Paso Rojo*

Of course, she was giving him to Bonnie, if Bonnie would comply with all these requirements, which the owner herself could not afford. This scenario is not as unusual as it might sound. I remember five other very similar chronic laminitis cases where I was called after the prior vet advised euthanasia. None of these cases were referred to me by the prior vet, and there were actually five different prior vets in those five cases. For this story I will just use Rojo's specific details.

Rojo was a grossly overweight 10-year-old Peruvian Paso gelding. He had very fine, clean, short pony legs, supporting a massive body and neck. His feet were actually very tough, but he had a history of repeated laminitis attacks and the white line separation was obvious and significant. He was not on Bute the day I saw him, and he was not real sore that day, but his problem was obvious. Bonnie wanted to know if he really needed all this expensive medication, feed, and supplements, or if she could simply put him on a diet to lose a couple hundred pounds. I agreed that would be a better plan than putting him to sleep.

I told Bonnie no grain, no alfalfa or clover hays, only grass hay (without seeds or leaves), and a muzzle if he was to be on pasture. Bonnie claimed to understand all that without seeming to pay much attention to me. She was anxious to take Rojo to a friend's barn and small paddock where there were no other horses, and she could totally control what he would eat.

Over the next three years, I was only called to see Rojo twice, both times for mild laminitis flare-ups. He had lost more than 100 pounds. The first time, the laminitis was triggered by very short clover in the paddock which Bonnie did not think was enough to need the muzzle. The second time, a year later, it was from a moderate amount of alfalfa leaves in what otherwise looked like grass hay. Both times he reportedly recovered in a few weeks with a short course of Bute and feed adjustments. I know there were also a couple other flare-ups I was not called to see, as Bonnie simply called to ask if she could pick up some Bute a couple other times.

Typically, her husband would be sent to pick up the Bute. About the fourth time they called for more Bute, I told them I had not seen Rojo in over a year, and I needed to see the horse occasionally in order to sell them the Bute. The husband said, "Well, what more can you do? She's spent a fortune on him at the XYZ Clinic. Nothing's worked, and she's promised to put him down this fall."

I refused to sell him the Bute. I hope no one reads this book and thinks you can treat laminitis with Bute without identifying and eliminating the feed triggers, proper trimming, and turnout. I use the minimum effective dose of Bute for as long as necessary for almost every case, but you MUST also identify and eliminate the triggers, which vary from case to case.

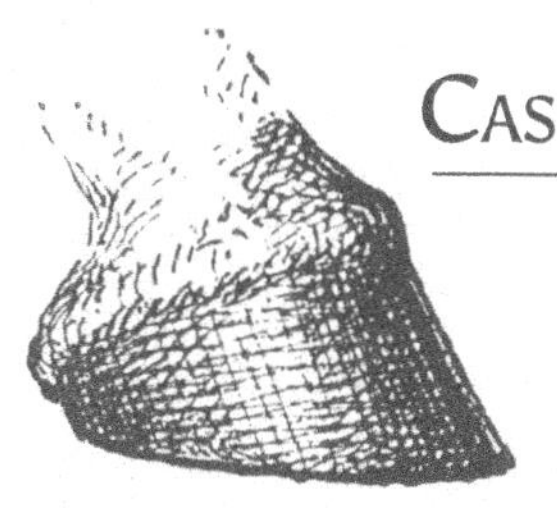

## Case Study

# "Harry" and "Di"

### *Two Nearly Identical Horses with Very Mild Cases of Acute Laminitis, but Delayed Diagnoses, One Fatal*

THESE TWO HORSES AND THEIR owners never met each other. However, the horses and their stories of very mild, unrecognized, acute laminitis were so similar, they need to be discussed together. Di recovered with minimal permanent damage, but Harry and his owner suffered his agonizing premature death from laminitis. Except for their difference in ages, these two horses could have been identical twins separated at birth but raised very differently.

Di was considered a Mustang by her owners because she had come through a Federal Bureau of Land Management capture and sale as a wild, untouched 6-year-old mare. It took several years of patience for her teenage sister owners to win her confidence. Harry was a registered American Quarter Horse with perfect manners and disposition, who might have been imprinted at birth by Dr. Robert M. Miller, the expert on natural horsemanship. These two horses lived about 50 miles apart at opposite ends of my practice territory. A judge would not have been able to separate the two horses in a halter class. They were virtually identical in size, conformation, and fitness, if not their early education.

I had been Harry's veterinarian for three years before he and Donna moved to Arizona in 2006. Two years later she called, on August 11, 2008. Donna was extremely upset, and she feared her best friend was in a near hopeless situation. Worst of all, she felt it may have been her fault for not recognizing the seriousness of his condition sooner.

I most clearly remember Donna always being present when I saw Harry, usually having a list of three to five questions every time I came for spring or fall vaccinations. Like all my clients, she had my cell phone number for questions if needed, but she never abused it. She did not live close to the stable, but she never missed a single veterinary visit for Harry, and she was always extremely polite, concerned, and thorough.

Harry was 19 years old, and I remembered him very well. He was an extremely pleasant horse to work with, an ideal trail horse for a suburban mother and housewife. Like Di, he was on the small side. They were not heavily muscled horses like many AQHA show ring specimens, and neither ever had any weight or serious soundness problems. Most people can learn to adjust their horse's feed simply by looking at his weight every day. That was never necessary for either Harry or Di. Both seemed to have a self-adjusting metabolism which maintained an ideal weight, regardless of the quality of the hay or the season of the year.

Harry was ridden barefoot from the time he was 6 until about age 12, when Donna was forced to shoe him because gravel on the trails near his stable repeatedly made his feet sore. The shoes were used with pads during the Illinois winters to prevent ice balls and later to protect his moderately thin soles from the hot summer Arizona ground.

Donna's distressing 30-minute phone conversation indicated Harry was boarding at a stable with about 25 other privately owned horses, each kept in an approximately 20-foot square pipe corral with a small awning for shade. Harry also had a stall with an attached 20' by 20' corral of hard-packed Arizona sand/clay. Donna drove to the stable most days, but the barn management was responsible for Harry's daily feed and care.

Donna related Harry had a very severe colic in July 2007, just two days before Donna and her husband had a vacation trip scheduled to visit their families in Illinois. The barn manager found Harry at 4:00 am lying down, sweating, bruised, and filthy from rolling. His impaction eventually responded to Banamine, Dipyrone, and a gallon of mineral oil. Two days later, Donna and her husband left for Illinois. Daily phone calls to her girlfriend, who was to keep an eye on Harry, and take him on a couple trail rides assured Donna that Harry was fine during her absence. But when Donna returned, Harry was showing some mild soreness that shifted from one front leg to the other. Donna's girlfriend said in retrospect he had seemed "a little slow and sluggish at the start of their rides, but that he quickly warmed up and was full of energy. He trotted and cantered easily whenever she let him move on." She thought this must be quite normal for a horse at age 19. No one suspected laminitis, and his mild and inconsistent "soreness" was attributed to age related arthritis. Donna gave him a little Bute before some of her rides. Donna still had not found a vet in Arizona she could call to ask her "silly little questions" without being charged several hundred dollars for a "trip charge, lameness exam, and digital radiographs." The colic treatment a few weeks earlier had already been like an extra month's board bill for a lady always on a budget.

After a few weeks of occasional Bute, Harry's "arthritis" was much better. He had been absolutely sound and on no Bute for a couple months. But in December 2007, Harry's farrier pointed out a white line separation. No one associated the slight separation with his colic five months earlier. The farrier said it appeared to be growing out and shod him the same as he always had.

The supposed "arthritis" returned in the spring of 2008 and was again treated with just an occasional dose of Bute. By summer, Harry was riding really well without any Bute at all. Donna remembered an especially great ride the week of July 4th, a year after his colic, when Harry had "the energy of a two-year-old." There had not been a hint of soreness for several months. On July 11th, Harry had a regularly scheduled reset of the shoes and summer pads. The very observant farrier did not see anything different when the shoes and pads were changed, but Harry was sore immediately thereafter. Donna suspected he had been trimmed just a bit short, and she gave him Bute for a few days while waiting for his feet to grow out a little. When this did not resolve the problem, she finally arranged the expensive veterinary appointment.

The veterinarian saw Harry for the recurring, persistent "arthritis" on July 28, two and a half weeks after the latest shoeing reset. Radiographs on the first visit showed 10 degrees of coffin bone rotation away from the right front hoof wall, and substantial sinking of the coffin bone within the left front hoof. The unsuspected laminitis had done a great deal of damage. I am sure Donna never neglected this horse. She and everyone else at the barn simply did not recognize the episodes of laminitis from the impaction the previous summer, then earlier that spring, and for 17 days between the shoeing and the eventual veterinary visit. Bute for the "arthritis" inadvertently half treated the mild disease which progressed to irreversible damage.

For over thirty years, I have maintained that mild laminitis is more likely to cause permanent damage, because it is so much harder to recognize and treat seriously before the damage gradually progresses. Generally, I have seen horses with sudden severe laminitis the first day I am called, and they virtually all have done very well, as long as the cause can be identified and eliminated, and the owner complies with the management and treatment advice.

My best advice for Donna on her August 11th phone call was to buy a rototiller and a hose to soften Harry's small corral. I didn't want it too deep, but soft moist ground could help make him more comfortable. Donna also had more sand brought in to get the right depth and cushion for the footing. Therapeutic shoes with a soft gel packing had been put on August 1st. I could not make any recommendations on those without a personal exam. Harry got steadily worse each day, until he was humanely euthanized a week later.

There are few options to treat chronic laminitis. It is dangerous to either soak or cold hose feet with Harry's advanced rotation and sinking. Softening a thin sole with too much water can easily allow the unstable coffin bone to penetrate the sole. Allowing a horse with a long toe and laminitis to walk puts too much strain on the toe laminae at break-over. The toe must be squared to ease break-over. Abscesses are also a constant threat with the separated laminae opening spaces, and the dropped coffin bone compressing the blood vessels beneath the coffin bone. These may be either sterile, necrotic abscesses from oxygen deprived cells dying, or infectious abscesses.

Generally, I believe in frequent trims by the farrier or vet. Barefoot is best, if his feet can tolerate it. I prefer to continually rasp back the toe and keep the heels low to realign the coffin bone with the front hoof wall and the ground when possible. Sometimes, especially talented farriers can apply a shoe which might do more good than harm, but I usually prefer barefoot. The minimum effective daily dose of Bute is critical to control inflammation and improve circulation. The strength of the digital pulse can be a good monitor for the dose of Bute needed along with gauging the horse's comfort while walking.

Eliminating the cause of laminitis is extremely important but it is hard for me to speculate at long distance in Harry's case. The impaction in July 2007 likely triggered his first undiagnosed laminitis. Since Harry never had a weight problem in Illinois, I don't suspect he developed one at age 19. He might have been developing Cushing's disease after the move, but I have never considered that a primary cause of laminitis. It certainly can predispose a horse to laminitis, requiring the owners to be more careful about feeds and weights. Diagnosing and treating Cushing's with pergolide can help, but it does not prevent laminitis when the other triggers are ignored.

The most common cause of mild laminitis relapses like Harry suffered is too-rich hay, grain, or pasture. I am sure Arizona hay is very different from Illinois hay. This does not require a laboratory analysis of the feed, and it does not mean the feed wasn't perfectly safe for the other horses. Individual horses can become sensitized to some feeds like alfalfa, so that they react much more quickly than non-sensitized horses.

Secondary factors could well be the small, hard surfaced corrals coupled with Harry's shoes and pads. Horses get significantly better circulation to their feet when turned out barefoot on soft ground. Stagnant circulation and the resulting inadequate oxygen to the laminae is the ultimate cause of laminar failure.

Di had a very similar laminitis, but a much happier ending. Di, who could have been Harry's identical twin sister, was considered by her owners to be a Mustang because she was raised wild on federal lands and went through a BLM auction after capture from the wild herds. In reality, her parents were likely western ranch horses turned loose to fend for themselves over the long winters. She looked identical to Harry but suffered from a lack of early domestication.

When her novice teenage sister owners were saddling Di for an early lesson about five years ago, she bolted and ran into a heavy gauge utility pole guy wire, leaving a 6 inch long by 2-inch-deep slice, just medial to her left eye.

This happened just as I was about to sit down to Easter Sunday dinner with my family, and I tried without success to get the owners to take Di to a clinic to repair what they were describing over the phone. They insisted, and I went reluctantly. The large wire cut was separated about an inch, and lateral muscles had pulled the entire eye an inch laterally. The guy wire had broken off a 1-inch section of the zygomatic arch bone, which I removed and discarded before suturing. She is totally normal, and much better behaved today. The scar can only be seen when she is fully shed out in the summer. The missing bone can easily be palpated and left not even a dimple on her forehead.

The sisters' mother called me March 15, 2013, to ask if she could pick up a tube of Bute. She said Di was a little sore footed after having her feet trimmed. This was not an unusual request, and knowing Di had never had a weight issue or any prior laminitis, I agreed to sell her the Bute without a visit. Di received 1 gram a day most days, until the mother called on March 28th to request more Bute. I declined to sell her a second tube until I paid a visit.

On examination, Di was maybe only 30 or 40 pounds overweight, but it was extremely obvious to me. Di was indeed sore footed just walking. I easily found a strong digital pulse which I had the mother and both sisters also feel. She was tender to the hoof testers over her toes, and even very light rapping on her front hoof walls caused her to flinch, but she ignored the tapping on her hind feet. I had the girls walk her on the blacktop and we could see how much it hurt her turning and torqueing the laminae on the pivot foot. I had the girls trot her on the blacktop, then repeated it after holding up one front foot for 30 seconds. The increased lameness in the foot she had to stand on was dramatic for everyone to see. I showed the mother and the girls all this so they could judge Di's recovery and adjust the minimum effective dose of Bute each day. As all those signs improved, I reduced the daily Bute dosage. I gave Di 2 grams of Bute IV and 3 cc of Lasix IV to treat the inflammation and edema in her feet. I then searched for the cause of her dramatic weight gain. She was getting no grain but had 24/7 access to a large round bale of hay. There was a very severe drought in 2012 in Illinois and hay was expensive. Normally, our best alfalfa hay is made into smaller square bales and sold for premium prices, but Di's round bale was extremely rich alfalfa. It was the cause of the weight gain and the laminitis. She shared it with four other horses who were not affected. We switched Di to mostly grass hay and limited the other horses' access to the alfalfa round bale. I left the girls 50 grams of Bute powder and instructed them to feed the minimum effective dose daily as Di's lameness improved.

When I went home, I emailed their mother some of my laminitis stories. Di was off Bute within two weeks of her diagnosis, and I did not need to make a return visit until July 1st, more than three months later. Di was extremely lame on her left front foot and I found an abscess at the toe which had a minimally separated white line from the two week delay in diagnosing acute laminitis in March. Trimming and drilling on the toe failed to release any fluid, but she was walking 50% better, so I applied iodine and Epsom salts covered with a diaper and duct tape to draw out the abscess. The girls and their farrier again did the follow up, and I only saw Di one more time on July 22nd to clean the abscess hole. Ten months later Di has had no further lameness issues. Because of her 2013 bout with laminitis, she has been sensitized to alfalfa, and she needed to be fed more carefully to prevent future flare-ups. Now she is sound for anything the girls want to do with her, from trails to barrel racing. I never met Harry's farrier, but I did speak with him on the phone after the horse was dead, and before writing up his case history. Like Di's farrier, I found him to be very intelligent and interested. Both have had to treat far too many foundered horses, and the often-conflicting advice they get from different veterinarians is a source of frustration.

My advice to both of them, is when you see something, say something. Both these horses were sore after trimming or shoeing because they had undetected acute laminitis at the time. It is likely the horses were not well behaved when required to stand on one foot with undetected laminitis. That would have been a better time to recognize, diagnose, and treat the disease.

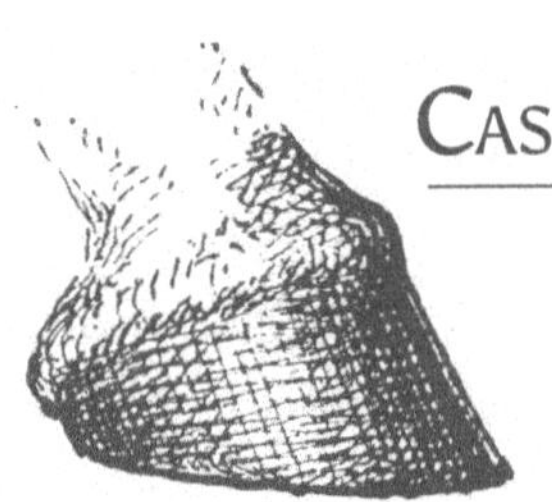

# Case Study

## "Charles"

### *Five Separate Flare Ups of Acute Laminitis in Eight Months... Fatal*

THIS IS CHRONOLOGICALLY THE LAST case I have written for this book, although other stories follow. It has haunted me for 25 years, but I did not write it up earlier because I could not figure out a way to tell the story without blaming my longest and most loyal client. Despite changing names, the facts were too unique to disguise. Each of these stories is unique. They are not composites or hypothetical stories. They come directly from my medical case records. Hopefully by reading all these stories, you will be prepared to recognize the most serious case earlier than we did here.

Gwen graduated high school a couple weeks after I graduated veterinary school. She was one of the first to call me after our hometown newspaper announced the opening of my brand new Equine Veterinary Service. She remained a very loyal client for more than 42 years of constant horse ownership.

Charles was a very nice 10-year-old AQHA gelding on whom I did a pre-purchase exam in April 1990. He was a beautifully trained fox hunter for Gwen. She planned to use him for her duties as a whipper-in for the fox hunt. That meant she would ride ahead of the field and help the huntsman control any wandering hounds who strayed too far afield from the pack. Charles was suitable in every respect for his intended purpose, a very sound, experienced, fit, and pleasant horse.

The fox hunt had a spring season in May 1990. Charles and Gwen very much enjoyed their role in helping to keep the pack of hounds focused. The job involved some barefoot running on the asphalt roads within the developing suburban hunt country. The horse I had pronounced fit for a life of fox hunting was sore on May 10th, after just his second hunt, because of fairly mild Grade II laminitis. Charles was not at all overweight. The spring pasture was just starting to grow faster, but I was more concerned with Charles' short feet. He had been trimmed by the regular farrier but left barefoot for better traction on the blacktop roads. The asphalt quickly wore his light-colored feet down dangerously short, and they were inflamed, more from abrasion than concussion or lush grass. While "road founder" is the horseman's term, it should be termed "road laminitis." Charles had not actually foundered. His coffin bone had neither rotated nor dropped within the hoof capsule. At the first visit, I prescribed a few days of Bute and a little pasture rest. He was running and playing in the pasture without Bute by the end of the week.

Gwen called back June 10th when Charles was sore again. After a month off, Gwen had him shod and resumed her duties as a whipper-in for the fox hunt pack. He was sore again two days after hunting very well. Again, his weight and feed issues seemed fine. The pasture still did not seem dangerous by itself, but Gwen admitted to a lot of running on the blacktop roads during the hunt. The shoes had protected his hooves from abrasion this time, but they did not protect from the concussion on blacktop. This flare-up was slightly more painful than the first time, so I removed Charles' shoes and had Gwen hose his feet and make a mud puddle for him, in addition to a moderate dose of Bute. According to Gwen, Charles looked great again the next day, but by the third day he was limping off his right front foot. He had developed an abscess under the coffin bone. This was a clear draining abscess, not the typical dark abscess from trapped dirt. The location, under the front rim of the coffin bone, indicated to me that very slight sinking of the coffin bone caused this seroma, which looks similar to a blood blister, but contains just serum. I treated it with iodine and Epsom salts and bandaged the hoof with a diaper and duct tape. We took him out of the mud lot because of the open wound. By June 19th, Gwen called to tell me he was running and bucking in the pasture again without any Bute.

Charles remained off Bute for several months and was ridden periodically around the farm that summer, between the spring and fall hunt seasons. Gwen called a third time for rather mild laminitis, but not caused by hard roads this time. Charles was on very good pasture every day, but the summer flies caused him to lose weight, so Gwen increased his grain. Charles was barefoot and he easily picked up both front feet for me. He had no separation at all in his white line. His soles were still concave. But he had a new fresh blood pattern visible in both front soles that exactly matched the shape and position of his coffin bones. Without any lameness visible to Gwen, low grade laminitis caused his coffin bones to drop over the past few weeks. The good pasture and grain to maintain his weight were a little more than his feet could tolerate.

This time his soles were too thin to tolerate mud puddles, and since the laminae were clearly under stress, I had to protect his now delicate feet. I squared his toes to ease his breakover and then applied iodine and Epsom salts, bandaged with diapers and duct tape, to his front feet. This is my version of Burney Chapman's famous "Sugardine" (sugar and iodine) dressing. If the feet are soft or thin, I use more salt to dry and toughen the sole. If horses have hard tough feet, I will use a damper solution to soften the foot. But softening the sole with inflamed laminae can be disastrous. If the expert farrier Burney Chapman had been available and affordable, this might have been a good time for expertly applied heart bar shoes.

I believe optimum circulation is necessary for rapid healing of laminitis, so I did not ask for stall confinement. I prefer the horse wander around a sand arena, but since Gwen did not have one at home he stayed on summer pasture, but without the grain meals. I always give the minimum effective daily dose of Bute, and Charles was again off Bute, walking fine, and out of his dressings within two weeks.

I had not done radiographs because the X-rays would not have changed my diagnosis or treatment. When I first X-rayed Charles' front feet on June 20th, there was only a very slight hint of movement of the right front coffin bone. I should have squared his toes at that point, but instead I used tape to secure frog support pads.

Charles did well the rest of the summer and was fox hunting again in August. My wife and I were in Europe the first week of September, and we had left my wife's horse, Surprise, with Gwen for the week. The Saturday morning before we returned home, Gwen found both Surprise and Charles in the barn with the grain tipped over, having eaten all they wanted. Someone had failed to double lock a large sliding barn door, and Prize, as he sometimes did at home, pushed the door to the side and found the grain barrel, like a mouse finds cheese. Both horses seemed fine all day Saturday and Sunday, so Gwen did not call my backup vet.

When Charles looked sore footed Monday morning (48 hours after getting into the grain), Gwen gave him some Bute before going to work. He was better that evening, and Surprise still looked fine to her. We were due home Tuesday but did not actually arrive until Wednesday. On Wednesday, I saw Charles and had him confined to a dry lot, wrapped his feet, and took away his grain. This was his third laminitis relapse in four months, and by far his most serious. Despite the Bute, he was still Grade II four days after getting the grain overload.

Three days later, he was worse instead of better. Then I walked his fence line and found a lot of deadly nightshade he had eaten through the fence when we confined him and restricted his intake. I consider this his fourth flare-up and the worst lameness all year—now Grade III and very serious. X-rays on September 14 still showed almost no rotation.

I removed his shoes again on September 14, and again I used the taped-on frog support pads. Charles reportedly again responded very well to the treatment and the Bute was gradually reduced.

My father had died of cancer October 10, 1990, after I took several trips to Kansas City. That may have been the reason Gwen did not want to bother me while Charles seemed to be recovering nicely. When I did see Charles again on October 17, despite a month of Gwen's "minimum effective" daily doses of Bute, and her frequent changing of the frog pads, X-rays showed Charles was rotated 13 degrees in the right front toe and 9 degrees in the left front toe. He had gotten far worse the past month without showing any dramatic pain.

We then had him shod with different frog pads, and the next X-rays, after shoeing, showed 11 degrees rotation in the right front side and 9 degrees in the left front. Three weeks later he was more painful, and when I removed his shoes and pads, his soles were as soft as Gwen's cheeks. I euthanized him on November 13, 1990.

For years, I silently blamed Gwen for not noticing the daily differences when he had very mild laminitis. After 25 years, I finally realized that while I have averaged about 30 cases of laminitis every year for over 42 years in the same Northern Illinois practice, this was Gwen's first case ever. In her 44 years owning and personally caring for her horses every day, Gwen has only had one other chronic laminitis in a Shetland pony that she bought years later for her young daughter. The pony did just fine with an occasional gram of Bute and a grazing muzzle when the pasture was growing rapidly. She managed him easily and usefully for years. Gwen has been an outstanding client and horse caretaker for over 42 years, and I have been proud to provide her veterinary care. I was the one who failed Gwen in 1990, by not teaching her all she needed to know about laminitis when she needed to know it. Laminitis was not a mysterious disease to me in 1990, and more research would not have saved Charles. He died because his owner was not adequately educated about the disease. I assumed she knew enough to make the judgment calls so necessary as the disease ebbs and flows day to day.

It can be very hard for the novice to notice changes with mild laminitis. You need to watch the horse very carefully and monitor the digital pulse often. Mild laminitis can, and will, kill a horse slowly over a month's time if the changes are not recognized and dealt with in a timely manner. Charles died needlessly, and it was mostly my fault. I was the expert with laminitis, and I should have driven out to Gwen's farm more often to check him myself. This book is my way of saying, "I'm sorry," and hopefully teaching thousands of other horse owners what they need to know to prevent their horses from dying of improperly treated laminitis, or laminitis diagnosed too late.

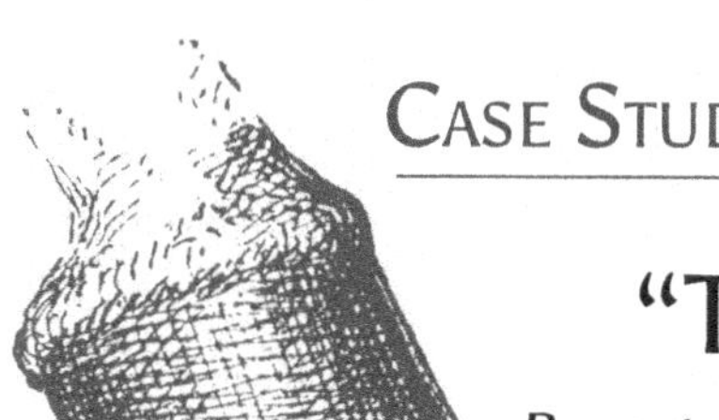

# Case Study

## "Taj" and "Liberty"

### *Repeated Laminitis Before Grazing Muzzles*

**UNLIKE SPIRIT AND DOTS, WHO** were both fully recovered from Grade III or IV acute laminitis within 1–3 days because they had extremely competent and compliant owners with sand arenas who each caught the disease on the first day of lameness, Taj and Liberty both had milder cases which were allowed to linger far too long, until I brought them to my own farm out of frustration. The differences in response to treatment were clear to me. And they need to be understood by the reader to prevent the same mistakes and deficiencies from damaging your horse. Taj was a 10-year-old black Arab gelding owned by, as far as I know, my only client to have had a six-page pictorial in *Playboy* magazine, although I did have a couple other retired Playboy Bunnies for clients. Mary and her friend stayed after my laminitis lecture as part of my horse health care class at the local junior college. They said Mary's horse had been lame on and off for months and was recently diagnosed with laminitis by a new vet. After my lecture, they thought I should see her horse. I saw him the next day.

Taj, a sharp looking black Arab, was not fat, but he did have a significant crest. He was very gimpy on both front feet, which had almost an inch too much toe for the size of the horse and his otherwise good-looking feet. He had an easily detectable digital pulse behind both front fetlocks, but not the rear fetlocks. I trimmed off some of the excess toe to ease breakover, but I found significant white line separation. This likely came from the long toes grabbing the ground and pulling against the weakened laminae the previous five or six weeks with untreated mild acute laminitis.

After administering Bute IV and trimming the feet we discussed the feed Taj was getting. His private pasture was still quite green in October, and there were large patches of clover. Grazing muzzles were not yet well designed and accepted in 1990. I showed Mary and her neighbor how to check the strength of the digital pulse and reviewed the lecture on laminitis I had given them in class the night before.

Taj was better the next day, and he was quickly down to just 1 gram of Bute a day. I saw him once a week and the girls reported his progress at class each week. He did not get off the Bute totally until the snow fell and covered the still green clover in November. He was fine all winter, but when the ground thawed in March the clover was the first to green up, and his laminitis returned. We had to treat him again with Bute.

Liberty was a teenaged gelding Belgium work horse. He came up lame the fourth or fifth summer I cared for him. He responded well to Bute and removal from the pasture. When he returned to the pasture the lameness recurred. We found areas of previously unsuspected clover. I moved him to my farm for several weeks, where he recovered just as uneventfully as Taj.

# ~SECTION X~

## Fatal Abscesses

## Case Study

# Lameness and Complicated Abscesses

### *Five Fatal (of 2,000) Hoof Abscesses*

IN HORSES, HOOF ABSCESSES ARE the most common cause of lameness in one leg, and easily the most common lameness I have been called to treat in my mostly backyard and small farm equine practice in NW suburban Chicago. A few times I've tried to count the number of hoof abscesses I have seen, and it was usually close to 50 per year. After 42 years in the same practice, I believe I've diagnosed and treated over 2,000 hoof abscesses, and five of them have died.

Sometimes the owners didn't notice a lameness, or thought the lameness was mild enough that it would probably go away on its own, without a vet visit. Given enough time, the abscess usually would migrate up the hoof wall and drain itself at the coronary band. Then the owner might call because they thought the horse cut his coronary band. Patiently waiting for this spontaneous cure can backfire, depending on the location of the abscess and the thickness of the hoof wall. Aside from unnecessarily lengthening the horse's days of pain, the abscess may undermine the entire sole before it opens at the bulb of the heel.

On two occasions I was called after an abscess remained unopened for months, to offer a third or fourth opinion. Both horses were euthanized because the spreading abscess had destroyed the sensitive toe laminae causing severe rotation of the coffin bone in a hind foot. In two other horses, an inadequately treated abscess caused the entire hoof to detach enough to slough off. I had one horse die from complications of a hoof abscess when an owner was unable to keep a hoof with a sole abscess clean and out of manure in his paddock. This was before I knew the benefits of diapering feet.

Typical abscesses are almost always found and cured with a combination of trimming the hoof, cleaning all dirty sole and white line areas with the rasp and hoof knife, using hoof testers to localize the most sensitive area, and then exploring all dark tracts to a sufficient depth until either necrotic pus is released, or the dark tract disappears. An experienced veterinarian can open and drain at least 90% of abscesses with a hoof knife. Done properly, there is rarely a drop of blood, and usually the horse is sound shortly after the pressure is released. The other 10% required that I visit a second, or occasionally a third time, over a period of a few days before I was able to locate and adequately drain the abscess tract.

I generally asked the owner/trainer to keep the hole cleaned and protected for about two weeks to allow the hoof to regrow from the inside out. In my first 15 years of practice, I would have the owner soak the hoof daily in a bucket of warm water and Epsom salts, and then pack the hole in the sole or white line with a small cotton ball. Over 20 years ago, I learned that disposable baby diapers, filled with iodine and Epsom salts, and secured with duct tape, are much more effective than daily bucket soaks and cotton balls. The concentration of iodine and Epsom salts can be adjusted depending on how dry or wet the hoof is. The goal is an optimum dampness; too wet is as bad as too dry.

While a diaper with iodine and Epsom salts will control the quality of the sole, Farrier's Formula strengthens the hoof wall. Horses with fragile or "shelly" hooves are predisposed to abscesses which are much more difficult to heal than if a horse has a high-quality hoof. My last 15 years in practice I noticed that a horse receiving Farrier's Formula for an extended time would grow a noticeably higher quality hoof wall, and I made Farrier's Formula part of the treatment for all my horses with fragile or "shelly" hooves.

One of the first two horses listed in paragraph 3 above was a Warm Blood mare who came in from the pasture one day limping like she had a broken leg. She was put on a month of stall rest, seen by three other vets over the next year, and then was still dead lame with a draining abscess at the frog. I put her to sleep the first night I was called, because I found an exposed coffin bone when I cleaned her necrotic abscess.

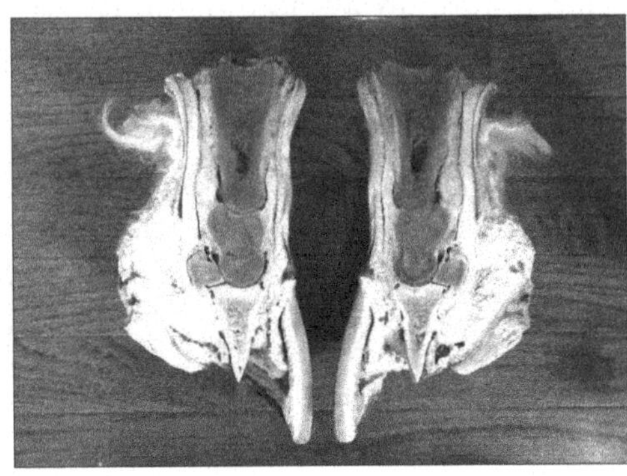

*Warm Blood Mare's Hoof Cut in Half*

The images here show her hoof cut in half and reveal the reason she wouldn't heal. The abscess began at the toe, but could not penetrate there and eventually worked its way about three quarters of the way up the inside hoof wall toward the coronary band and underneath the sole to the bulb of the heel. This horse had been on Farrier's Formula the entire year she was confined in a stall, which gave her an incredibly high-quality hoof wall.

A horse owner should suspect an abscess when his or her animal is lame in one foot. Adequate drainage, often combined with diapers containing Epson salts and iodine, can prevent the infection from causing irreversible damage.

# ~SECTION XI~

## Off the Track Thoroughbreds

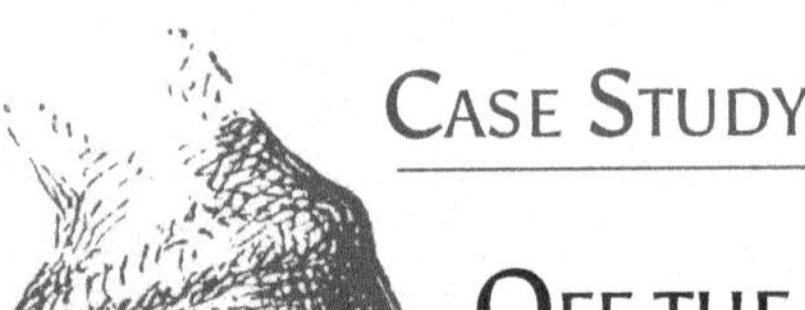

## Case Study

# Off the Track Thoroughbreds

### *"Casey," "Tiger," "Splash," "Buster," & "Milwaukee Wolf"*

OFF THE TRACK THOROUGHBREDS USUALLY live with some degree of chronic arthritis, which will flare-up from time to time when they jump, do dressage, or just play in the field. It can be very easy for even very experienced vets to miss mild acute laminitis in horses that have another periodic minor lameness.

Some academics will tell you this is not "evidence-based medicine" because I do not have double blind trials to support my theory of vasocompression rather than vasoconstriction. I have a 42-year clinical trial, treating over 1,200 real clinical cases of acute laminitis as vasocompression, while about two thirds of veterinarians have been treating it as vasoconstriction. I welcome a comparison of my 2% death rate to the nationally published 6% death rate, which might include about 1/3 of vets treating as I do and having a similar 2–3% death rate, while the other 2/3 treating vasoconstriction may have an 8–10% death rate. This equates to a 3 to 5 times greater risk for your horse to die.

There are also two published studies of acute laminitis treated on the farm by academic oriented vets. These two studies, done to investigate possible links between Cushing's disease and prednisolone to 102 cases of laminitis, each showed 25% laminitis death rates over the course of the studies. Those 102 horses were not hospitalized. Finally, there is the devastating 50% death rate published several times by certain hospitals. Such a high death rate is only partly due to sicker and more seriously injured horses in the hospitals than non-hospitalized horses. It is also due to the stall confinement, drug treatment of presumed vasocompression with vasodilators, and "therapeutic shoes," favored in hospitals. It might also be due to a higher percentage of Thoroughbreds and competition Quarter Horses in hospitals than I see in my suburban, mostly backyard, horse practice.

Off the track Thoroughbreds are usually the opposite feeding challenge of the easy keeper equine metabolic syndrome (EMS), or insulin resistant (IR), fat ponies that are constantly prone to laminitis flare ups. Most horse people know the great Thoroughbreds Secretariat and Barbaro were euthanized due to the uncontrollable pain of severe laminitis. Many horse people do not realize that the Thoroughbred racing magazines have reported the euthanasia, due to laminitis, of additional famous retired thoroughbred champions almost every week for decades. These are usually retired stallions and mares who have lived on Kentucky Bluegrass breeding farms for years, after winning hundreds of thousands of dollars at the racetracks. They are typically on the finest farms in the world and visited by the best veterinarians any day of the year. These great racehorses are most often owned by wealthy people who are willing to spend any amount of money to keep their best ever retired famous champions healthy and happy until they die of old age.

I have seen many gruesome slideshows at the national laminitis symposia, given by expert Lexington veterinarians who have gone to extremes attempting to salvage these mangled hoof disasters. Given the resources available to these owners, why are the horses being euthanized for laminitis, which I claim throughout this book is so easy to treat?

Four horses in this section, treated in 2010 and 2011, demonstrate again the dramatic difference between acute laminitis and the complications of chronic laminitis. My two recent laminitis disasters, Splash and Buster, were both off the track Thoroughbreds who died not because of their acute laminitis, but because they were not diagnosed and properly treated. While at the same time, twenty miles away, Tiger and Casey were both having repeated bouts of acute laminitis which were quickly recognized and very effectively treated. Neither Tiger nor Casey suffered any laminar damage. Luck and the "mysterious nature of laminitis" had absolutely nothing to do with which two horses quickly recovered, and the other two that had to be euthanized after long, painful, and expensive struggles.

Splash and Buster, whose wonderful owners did everything possible to save their horses' lives, did not receive the help they needed at the start of the disease, when the laminitis was very mild, and they could have been fully cured.

Retired, off-the-track Thoroughbreds make up less than 5% of my patients, but I dealt with enough of them over 42 years practicing equine medicine in the Chicago suburbs surrounding Arlington Park to know that they are distinctly different from the majority of backyard horses. The laminitis in four of the six horses in this section happened in my 37th and 38th years in the same private practice. The reasons for the vastly different outcomes are extremely important and obvious to me. The differences must be understood by all who own and care for horses; if they want to be prepared to prevent horrible suffering and save their own horse's life someday.

## Case Study

# "Casey"

### *Increased Feed Requirements in Older Horses Increases the Risk of Laminitis*

CASEY WAS A 33-YEAR-OLD retired eventer and fox hunter, who had been a patient of mine since he was purchased as a 4-year-old for Sally, a high school girl. Casey had some Thoroughbred breeding, but a 1/4 Percheron or Shire cross gives him much more substance than any horse that ever raced for a living. Casey is the only horse in this group who was not a racetrack Thoroughbred. When I did Casey's pre-purchase exam in 1984, he had no evidence of any lameness, and he had no sensitivity to my hoof testers. Unlike most Thoroughbreds, Casey always had large, round, very tough hooves. Shortly after he was purchased, Casey shed very thick soles in both front hooves without showing evidence of major infections, inflammation, or abscesses.

Sally trained and rode Casey through her college and early adult years. When she married and started raising her own three children closer to the city, her time to visit and ride Casey in the countryside became very limited. Casey stayed at the home of Sally's parents until her mother passed in 1998. Sally's widowed father sold their home, and Casey moved to a retirement farm at age 20. I continued to be his vet for several more years at that farm, until he moved to a second retirement farm 100 miles further into the country at age 25.

Sally and her sister brought Casey to my farm in 2008, at age 28, when the retirement farm manager reported that Casey was ready to be put to sleep. That day, Casey was pathetically close to 100 pounds underweight because he needed much more grain than he had been receiving.

I fed Casey eight pounds (two large coffee cans) of my grain mix twice a day, and our very good pasture. He probably gained 25 pounds the first week, and another 25 pounds the second week. Within a month his weight was where I wanted it, so I backed off the grain to what I thought would be a reasonable maintenance level. Casey quickly started losing weight again. Over the five years he was with us, Casey needed about eight pounds of mixed grain (including Senior feed, cracked corn, complete pellets, and sweet feed) twice a day to maintain his weight. When he was younger and working hard, he never needed that much grain. With both Casey and Tiger, it was a challenge to keep their weight looking good in the summer of 2011, and we fed what to most horse owners would consider excessive grain to both horses.

Horses on our farm lived outside 24 hours a day, about 350 days a year. They had a comfortable run-in shed for wind and rain. We opened the barn door twice a day, they came into stalls to be fed grain separately. Casey had acute laminitis once in May 2010, three separate times in May, June, and August 2011, and again in January 2012. He recovered quickly every time. His worst bout with acute laminitis was May 2011 when the grass was especially lush and growing fast. That time it lasted almost ten days, but each of the other four episodes resolved in less than five days. For the past three years, Casey has only been ridden for about ten minutes, two or three times a year by Sally or my high school aged son. He always looked sound walking and trotting around the pasture. But with an acute laminitis attack he would be very obviously sore-footed while walking out of his stall after eating his grain. He then would look fine in the summer, walking around the pasture grazing all day, and be fine when he walked back in for his next grain meal. In the winter, with frozen ground and no flies, he would not walk nearly as much.

It was not the grain which made Casey noticeably sore right after eating, but the length of time he was left in the stall. Our barn had railroad tie floors and when the horses were not staying in overnight, we would use a little straw on the floors. A horse with even mild inflammation and edema in his feet from laminitis will get stagnant circulation to his laminae standing in a stall on hardwood floors for an hour without frog pressure. The soreness is especially obvious the first couple steps when he has to pivot to make a left turn leaving the stall. By the time he is back in the pasture, the frog pressure has the blood in his feet moving again and the soreness disappears. This was reported with Barbaro, but apparently the significance was not appreciated at his hospital. I also saw it and wrote about it with Surprise, Jet, M.J., Breeze, and Wolf. It is an important clue to acute laminitis that should not be ignored.

Six months later, Casey was still sore coming out of his stall if he was in too long after eating. He needed the eight pounds of grain twice a day to hold his weight. I also added 1 gram of Bute powder and 1 scoop of Cosequin to his morning feed. It was extremely difficult to tell how much of his soreness might be due to laminitis and how much was age related arthritis. I could not feel an increased digital pulse, and he walked quite well once he was back out of the barn.

After one more summer of progressively worsening arthritis, it became obvious that rapidly developing and painful bone spurs on his left knee were causing most of Casey's lameness. The daily Bute for arthritis pain can interfere with the normal repair of cartilage, leading to the bone spurs. We did not feel it fair to make Casey go through another winter and euthanized him in October 2013, at age 33. It was a very good decision because 2013–14 was as bitter a winter as I ever saw in over 60 years in Chicago. I had 19 horses that died or were euthanized from January to June 2014, of whom, 14 were in their 30s.

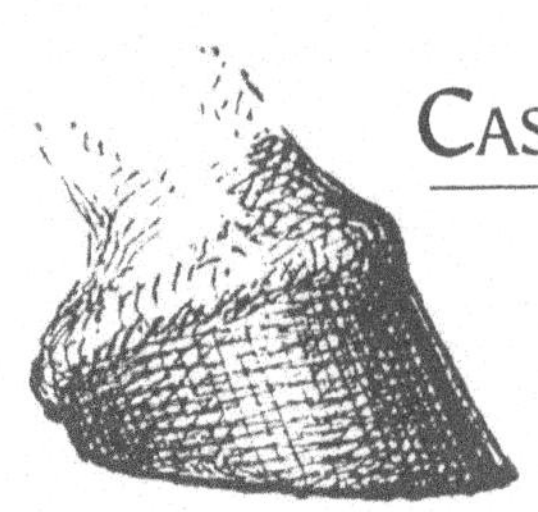

## Case Study

# "Arctic Tiger"

### *Flat Soles Increase the Risk of Recurrent Laminitis*

IN THE THREE MONTHS TIGER was on our farm (July to September 2011) he had two separate bouts of acute laminitis showing the same signs as Casey. However, Tiger had a much flatter sole than Casey, and with his fly sensitivity it was even harder to keep Tiger's ribs covered when turned out in the summer months. With Tiger I had to use a little more Bute and put more straw in his stall because of his flatter sole, his significantly weaker hooves, and a shorter window of opportunity to treat the acute laminitis before risking permanent damage to his higher risk feet.

I gave Tiger 2 grams of Bute just once in July and twice in September. With Casey, I only used 2 grams of Bute one time during his episode in May 2011. For the other four episodes, Casey received no Bute at all. Neither horse had to wear a muzzle, because reducing the large amounts of grain was enough to resolve the flare ups, without having to limit their pasture.

If either Tiger or Casey had been fat they would have needed longer treatment, and they certainly would not have been getting any grain from me. Every horse is an individual and there are many factors which contribute to the laminitis and possible effective treatments such as Bute. I much prefer to use lower drug dosages if I can reverse the course of the disease with other management.

Many of my clients think a stall for a horse is like offering a person eight hours of sleep in a good bed every night. I believe time outs, family dinner, and good sleep are effective and beneficial for raising children, but I do not believe stalls are beneficial for acute laminitis.

In preparing this report I flipped through my case records and found ten additional retired Thoroughbreds with laminitis in the past ten years. Seven of those ten required just one visit to diagnose, explain the cause and begin treatment of their laminitis. The other three required a second visit, and all recovered with no damage, because their owners called before any damage was done. Had their owners ignored the early mild lameness or received bad advice, it is very possible several of them would have suffered the same end as Splash and Buster.

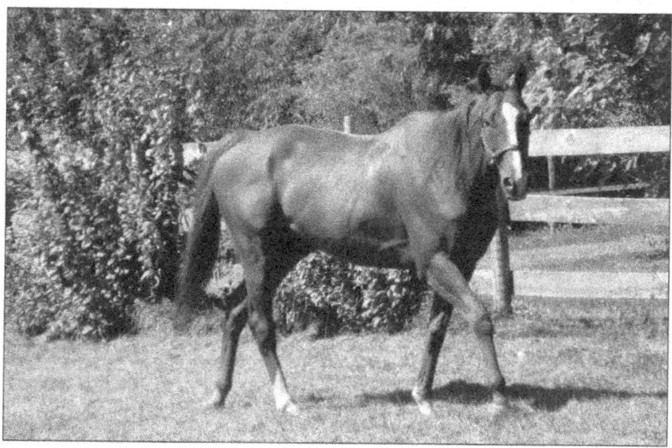

*Arctic Tiger*

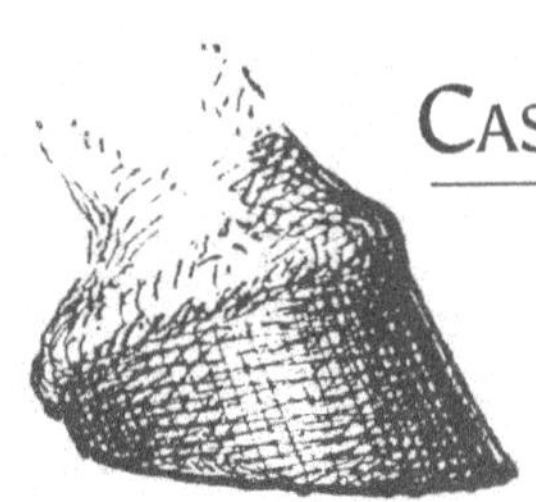

CASE STUDY

# "World Class Splash"

## *Best Care in the World, But Too Late*

TWO THOROUGHBREDS DIED IN 2011 because I did not get to them soon enough. As I wrote in the September 1997 *American Farrier's Journal* (1), "saving the life of a horse whose feet are collapsing due to uncontrolled chronic laminitis might be the most difficult and unrewarding job asked of veterinarians and farriers." After 19 additional years' experience, I would add owners and caretakers to those who have the hard job. The owners of Splash and Buster put more than ten hours of very hard work into trying to save their horses for every one of mine. Susie and Irene are my heroes for their efforts trying to save Splash and Buster.

World Class Splash was a very much loved 20-year-old gelding who still holds the track record at Arlington Park for a mile by a 3-year-old on the turf course. He had been placed by his trainer, J. R. Smith, in an ideal retirement situation at the age of seven, with Susie, a very classy and experienced horse loving grandmother. Susie, amazingly active and healthy into her 70s, personally fed Splash, groomed him, turned him out in her beautiful 5-acre pasture, cleaned his immaculate stall, and loved him every day. He shared his perfect barn and pasture with just one Morgan gelding. Susie rode Splash in the dressage ring and on the trails for 13 years. Susie's retired professional husband was the full-time grounds keeper, and the barn, pastures, and fences were perfect. No horse could ever hope for a better home than Splash had for his last 13 years.

Unfortunately, Susie and Splash lived 20 miles from me and used two other veterinarians in their first 12 happy years together. When Susie first noticed that Splash was off in July 2010, she called her then current vet, a full-time equine veterinarian with ten years' experience. With digital X-rays on July 17th, she ruled out laminitis and diagnosed Splash with "foot soreness from stomping flies on the hard summer pasture." The vet advised shoes and fly spray or leg wraps. I have made this same diagnosis a number of times when the ground gets very hard from lack of rain and the flies are bad. Susie had Splash shod and rode him several times a week the next month, but when he was still not quite right, Susie had the vet back out on August 16th. This time the digital X-rays showed 6 degrees of new rotation of the coffin bone in both front feet. Different therapeutic shoes were advised, and Splash was confined to his stall for the next three weeks.

Splash got steadily worse while confined to his stall after the second shoeing, and Susie was referred by a friend to a "natural" horse trimmer. She pulled the shoes and trimmed the feet, which gave some immediate relief. The new trimmer was a client of mine and knew I believed in allowing a horse with acute laminitis to be turned out. She suggested Susie get a second opinion from me.

I saw Splash for the first time that same day, September 7, 2010. Unfortunately, that was almost eight weeks after Splash's soreness had started. He had very fragile feet, with thin, brittle walls, a separated white line, and a dropped sole. Susie's husband had crushed limestone packed around both barn doors to prevent mud from the roof rain runoff. I pointed out how abrasive that was to Splash's fragile hoof walls and the next day there were much softer wood chips outside the barn doors. The pasture was thick and about 8" long. I suggested 4" would be better. It was mowed that afternoon. The Morgan horse was much heavier than Splash with a substantial crest to his neck. I advised muzzles for both horses. They bought and started using grazing muzzles that same day. A few days later I walked the newly mowed pasture and found quite a few thick clover patches, which I believe is a very common laminitis trigger. Her husband sprayed and killed the clover within a few days. I suggested boots or slippers for Splash's brittle and sore feet. They bought and used both. They bought memory foam from a mattress company to cut special inserts for the boots. They quickly complied with almost every suggestion I made to help Splash.

The one suggestion Susie never accepted was to leave Splash outside at night. She had to tuck him in every night to lie down and sleep in his beautiful soft and deep stall. He also had an ideal three-sided lean-to which was bedded like a stall for daytime use, but Susie was never comfortable letting him stay out at night. We know that walking is better for circulation than standing or lying in a box stall, but I never won that argument.

For almost a year, Susie struggled to save Splash. Before we could grow good hoof wall, Splash's coffin bones dropped and crushed the circulation between the coffin bones and soles. He developed necrotic abscesses under both coffin bones. Wrapping his feet with diapers and duct tape kept them much cleaner than the boots and slippers. It was very difficult to change the hoof bandages every day, as Splash could usually not stand on three feet for more than a few seconds.

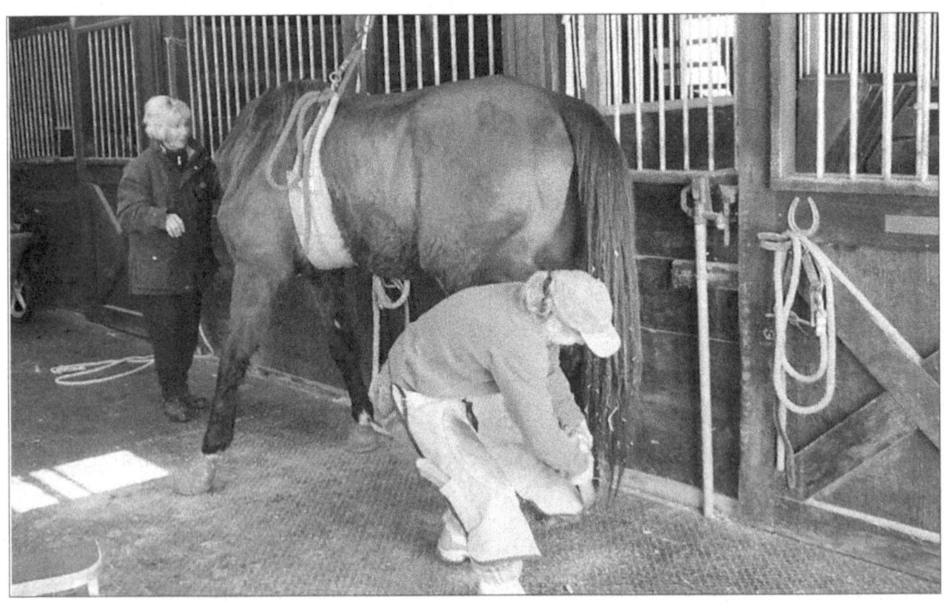

*World Class Splash*

Often, Susie would change his bandages while Splash would lay on his side. He would never do that for me, so when I came three or four times a month to assess his progress and debride the necrotic soles, we would hold Splash up with an 8" wide girth and a block and tackle hung from the barn joist. Splash was as cooperative as any patient in such pain could be. He never lost his appetite, and his will to live and appreciation for Susie's incredible efforts were obvious to everyone who tried to save him. Besides Susie and me, there were five additional experienced and dedicated farriers and horse owners/clients who came to help many times over the course of the year.

Splash eventually grew outstanding hoof walls, thanks mainly to Farrier's Formula, and localized intense light therapy. But we were never able to fully close the holes in his soles. The blood supply was so damaged that he lost a significant portion of one coffin bone to avascular necrosis. There was frequently significant progress, which we could all see, but then the setbacks would come. In my 42 years, no horse and owner ever tried harder than Splash and Susie, but after a year we had to admit defeat and let him go.

Splash's last two setbacks came when the farrier thought his feet were looking so good that he advised turning him out without bandages on his feet. Within a few days the soles were in very bad shape again. The final insult happened when another vet was called for a fifth set of digital X-rays to assess Splash's progress. This was the first time that particular younger vet had seen Splash, and she told Susie how dangerous daily Bute was (after a year on the minimum effective daily dose) and that he should be switched to firocoxib, a newer, more expensive, and supposedly safer and more selective NSAID.

Susie called three days after switching to firocoxib without my knowledge to tell me she had not been able to get Splash out of his stall since the other vet had told her to stop the Bute. Restarting the Bute at that point only made his pain more tolerable so he could get out to his pasture. It was beyond any further hope that he still might heal.

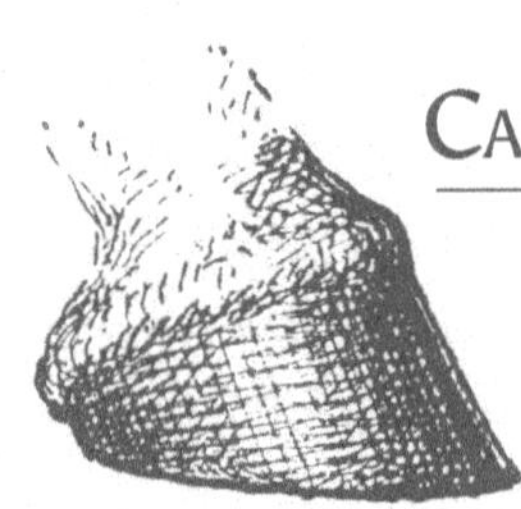

## Case Study

# "Buster"

### *Another Poor Veterinarian Client Relationship*

VETERINARY MEDICINE IS NOT ONLY a blend of art and science, but it is also a mixture of private business and public service. There also has to be a blend of decision making and diplomacy as you try to convince the owner what would give his horse the best chance for recovery, when recovery is a reasonable possibility. When presenting the treatment options, the owners often understand the odds best if you say the horse has an 80% chance for recovery or a 50% chance. Some owners need at least an 80% chance before they will go forward, while other owners will keep trying when there is only a 2% chance. The odds will change day to day as different complications develop. While Buster was riding the roller coaster of severe laminitis complications, Irene asked me one day, "Is this what recovery looks like?"

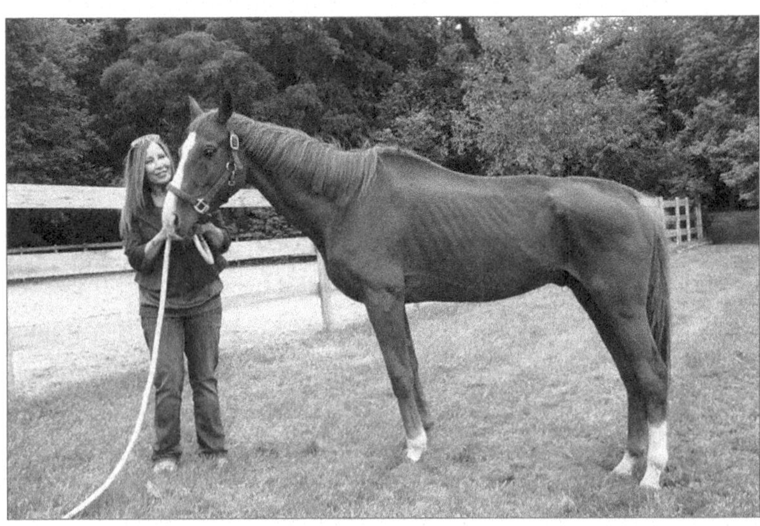

*Buster*

Irene was a retired bank VP who had never personally cared for a horse before assuming a huge responsibility trying to save Buster's life. She learned more in three months than many clients learn in thirty years. I was incredibly proud of the effort she and Susie put into trying to save Buster after Splash was gone. Buster was kept at a relative's five-acre home on the side of a ravine with two other fat horses. I had been called to the brother-in-law's barn three times the previous four years. They knew very little about keeping horses. All three were apparently "give away" free horses. The horses were obviously fed as a group every day, but I was only called for injuries or severe abscess type lameness. They probably wormed the horses occasionally, but I was never asked to vaccinate them.

The barn was at the bottom of a small but steep ravine. They would bring the injured horse up the side of the hill for me. I could not drive down to the barn. I had a hip replaced in 2007 and a triple bypass in 2010, so, in my mid-60s, I had little interest in walking down and climbing back up to my truck multiple times for drugs and supplies. Each time I treated one of the injuries or abscesses, the brother-in-law would jokingly say, "Well, I sure hope I don't have to see you again anytime soon," as he paid the $60 or $70 to treat the latest injury. I silently agreed, because there was no real veterinarian-client-patient relationship, and I would have been happy if they had called someone else for their next horse injury. Nevertheless, I went when they called because of my public duty.

The first week in September 2011, they called because Buster could not walk. They couldn't get him out of the barn. I happened to have a younger vet riding with me that day. Buster was our last stop, about 7 pm the same day they had called. It was starting to get dark when we arrived, and he was not at the top of the hill by the house. The wife insisted he could not walk out of the barn. We went down the side of the ravine. Buster was skin and bones, emaciated, with Grade IV laminitis. The other two horses were fat. Most likely it was the kids' job to feed the horses every day, and Buster was in desperate condition before the parents noticed. None of them had ever heard of laminitis. They thought his lameness was another abscess, which I had treated once a year or two earlier. He had also had an abscess blow out the coronary band a few times and get better on his own, saving the vet's fee. There was evidence of a recent blowout on one front hoof that I had not been called to see. Buster had the throbbing pulse of laminitis in all four feet.

We forced Buster out of the barn and started to hose his feet. We could not pick up either front foot for more than a couple seconds. I held my breath and got my truck down the gravel road to give him injections of Bute and Lasix. He got a little relief as we started walking him. There was not a level spot of grass anywhere to walk on. The barn really was at the bottom of a ravine on a rocky glacier hillside. I told them how serious it was, and that the horse's only chance was to take him to a neighbor who had an outstanding barn, sand arena, pasture, and knowledgeable experience a half mile up the road. I drove over to ask the experienced clients for permission. Not even knowing the folks down the road, they immediately agreed to my plan. The sister-in-law told us the horse could never walk that far. The other vet walked him down the road while I drove behind him with my headlights and flashers as it was getting rather dark on the road. We treated Buster there the next three days. When we could lift a foot for a few more seconds the next day, it turned out Buster had two draining abscesses in each front foot, in addition to the Grade IV laminitis.

We left him out in the sand arena with a flake of grass hay in each corner, and he wandered from corner to corner the next three days, when he wasn't flat on his side. I checked his progress and treated his feet each day, Tuesday through Friday, and my bill for the four visits and the Bute and furosemide was about $275. The man then said his sister-in-law owned Buster, and she would be out to see him on Saturday, and he would get me a check. The absentee ownership was news to me, but I told him to have her call me if Buster was her horse.

She did not call until the next Friday. Bubba never told her I asked her to call me. He thought it was way too much money for a pathetic looking old horse that was probably going to die anyway. She finally called on her own when the horse started getting much worse again after another week without seeing a vet.

Irene was the opposite of her brother-in-law, and she learned more about horses the next three months than I would have thought possible. She had only been the "owner" of Buster because her 90-year-old father had enjoyed going to the races, and he later enjoyed coming out to feed Buster carrots on occasion. For this, Irene subsidized Buster's feed costs. Her father had died six months earlier, but Irene continued to leave checks for "her dad's horse" when she and her husband visited his brother. The first time I met Irene, she told me that she would never give up on an animal. She told me about paying a $300 dental bill for a feral cat in the neighborhood.

After a couple weeks changing bandages and treating abscesses at the neighbor's home, Irene was being pressured by her brother and sister-in-law to bring Buster home. Not only would it be much harder for me to monitor him at the bottom of the ravine, but it would be much more difficult for Buster to walk around there. Walking promotes circulation to the feet, and the best possible circulation would be needed to heal both his laminitis and abscesses. The laminitis was responding much better than the multiple abscesses, which kept rupturing at the coronet, and proved very difficult to fully drain at the sole or the white line.

After just three or four days back home, it was obvious to Irene how much more difficult it was to treat him there. I then contacted another very experienced client who ran an outstanding boarding stable. She agreed to take on Buster. His laminitis was far better by then, but the abscesses still needed daily treatments. Irene paid her extra to soak Buster's abscesses and change his bandages every day. I had lightly floated Buster's teeth about a week after Irene assumed responsibility for his daily care, but he still was not gaining enough weight. While the laminitis was no longer an imminent danger, feeding him to regain weight while treating laminitis was a real challenge. A very experienced Master Equine Dentist (MED) visited Buster to cut off some badly overgrown molars that had been limiting his chewing motion for years. We were all shocked to see four very large and ugly ulcers on Buster's tongue and inner cheeks. It was unclear how much of the ulcers had been caused by sharp teeth and how much was a result of a month of daily Bute. If stress causes ulcers in Thoroughbreds, Buster was certainly under severe stress from his now month-long ordeal.

After three or four weeks at the boarding stable, Buster was on a plateau. His laminitis was gone, but the abscesses in both front feet continued to flare up and drain. Putting any weight on him was extremely difficult—his whispered nickname among the other sympathetic boarders was "Bones." He was spending far more time in his stall than I liked. Splash had been gone about a month and I asked Susie if she would consider allowing Irene and Buster to move to her home. Irene and Susie had never met each other, but they became fast friends and Buster had two of the best nurses anyone could ever hope for his last month while they fought the hoof infections.

Like Splash, Buster grew far better hoof wall within two months on Farrier's Formula, but the holes in the soles never fully healed. His walls were so thick that the infections repeatedly worked their way up and ruptured at the coronary band. I drilled holes in the walls and Irene flushed them with iodine daily. We fed Splash oral antibiotics, but the antibiotic can only go where the blood flows. And we know the blood supply to his sole was crushed. That is a big reason why the soles would not fully heal for either Splash or Buster. Blood vessels can regenerate over time, if we keep the pressure off and infection out. Buster did gain weight, and his oral ulcers were about 75% smaller after he had been at Susie's a couple weeks. I'm sure Buster felt he had already died, and this third new farm really was heaven. The farrier recommended an antifungal soak. I felt it was worth a try.

We were used to dealing with 1-inch horizontal separations of his coronary band from time to time, but three days after the 45-minute antifungal soak Buster's coronary band was separated 3⁄4 of the way around the hoof. I have only seen two horses slough a hoof and I did not want Buster to be the third. Amazingly, he was walking very well on that very nearly sloughed hoof, but I was sure that if he trotted, or even turned fast, it would fall off. Everyone had tried their best, but we had to put him to sleep that day.

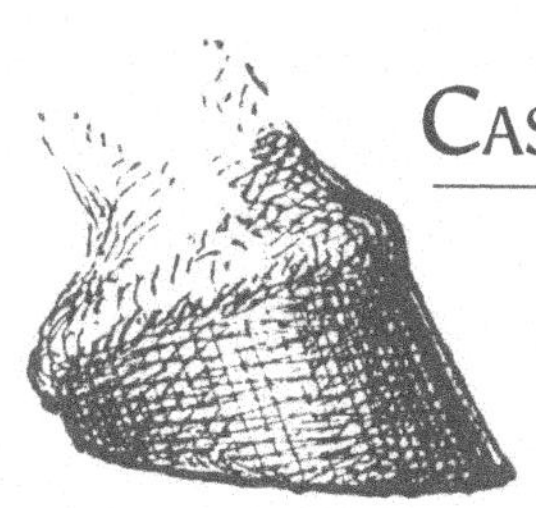

# CASE STUDY

## "MILWAUKEE WOLF"

### *Post-Doctorate Lessons in Repeated, Very Hard to Recognize, Acute Laminitis (Now Called SubClinical Laminitis)*

MILWAUKEE WOLF WAS A STRIKING 3-year-old Thoroughbred colt when I was asked to castrate him on June 26, 2010. He had just arrived on my client's farm in the countryside that catered to horses who needed a break from the racetrack. Trudy was 70, a retired racetrack trainer, and she handled all the farm chores for eight to ten turnouts by herself! Wolf stood perfectly for me with Trudy on the lead shank. I used just a short acting tranquilizer and local anesthetic for the standing castration, with no twitch or even a lip chain. It could not have gone smoother. Wolf 's confidence, attitude, barn manners, conformation, and pleasant disposition made such an immediate impression on me that day that I asked Trudy to call me if the owner wanted a good home for this horse when he was finished racing. Unfortunately, Wolf developed a swelling the next day which I feared might be a hernia. He got a quick trip to the hospital, where I watched a better surgeon easily resolve a simple hematoma under general anesthesia, which had intimidated me. Wolf was then turned out for a year to let his bowed tendon heal, before he returned to the racetrack. I had palpated the tendon before gelding him, and I felt it was quite insignificant compared to the bowed tendons I was used to seeing from my 20 years racing Standardbreds. There was no pain or tenderness on palpation, and very minor scar tissue was present. He seemed sound enough to me to have raced the day I castrated him.

On July 14, 2013, I received the call from Trudy asking me if I remembered the colt I had gelded three years earlier. I absolutely remembered Wolf. I still believed, without having seen him in three years, that with his disposition and conformation, he would be an outstanding trail, pleasure, show, or fox hunter for my wife. I learned from Wolf 's full racing record that he had raced six times as a 2-year-old and four more times at three before his actual third birthday. All ten races, before I first saw him, had been over his first winter as a baby in Florida. Wolf looked fabulous to me despite this intense early start at the races for a previous owner and trainer, before being claimed after his tenth race by the Illinois owner and trainer. He was very mature despite his small size, barely 15 hands at the time. He looked ready for either a show ring or the starting gate. His tendon issue seemed very minor to me. He simply made a huge impression on me as a very likely sweet, smart, and stylish riding horse when his racing career was over.

Trudy told me the trainer and the vet at the racetrack felt Wolf needed another year of turnout because the tendon was bothering him again. Wolf's owner believed he had raced enough. He was the only horse Barry, more a racing fan than horse owner, had ever owned. "Wolfie" had paid for his three years of racing out of his Chicago purse winnings, and Barry did not want to risk hurting him by bringing him back to the races again at age 7. Finding a good home was most important to Barry. My wife (who actually prefers not to ride Thoroughbreds) reluctantly agreed to check out the horse with me at the track the next day. She had just spent two years starting a young Paint horse, and she was not looking for another project. One good horse at a time was enough for her.

Wolf looked and behaved as well at Arlington Park as I had remembered him three years earlier. We met Barry for the first time, and everyone agreed it was time for Wolf to change careers at age 6. The tendon still did not look or feel any different to me than it had three years earlier. Most importantly to me, there was not a hint of arthritis in his ankles or knees despite 38 races! This horse's conformation really had proven to be as good as I thought three years earlier. He was an extremely clean legged retired racehorse.

We took Wolf home on July 17th, thinking I would put a soft gel cast on the tendon to allow it time to stabilize before asking my wife to start riding him lightly around our farm in about a month. When we got him off the trailer at our farm, he immediately started acting like a wild, tough racehorse. My wife much prefers quieter crossbreds to hot Thoroughbreds, and she did not like the way he started prancing and snorting in his new environment away from the racetrack routine. I put him in a stall the first night with a soft cast on the tendon. Since he had been walking absolutely sound, I put him in a 50-foot grass round pen the next day. I hoped he would quickly settle down and wander about the round pen. Instead, he ran and trotted in circles, without a hint of lameness. I was worried he might aggravate the tendon, but when I changed the soft cast several days later there was absolutely no change in the tendon, and still no lameness or tenderness.

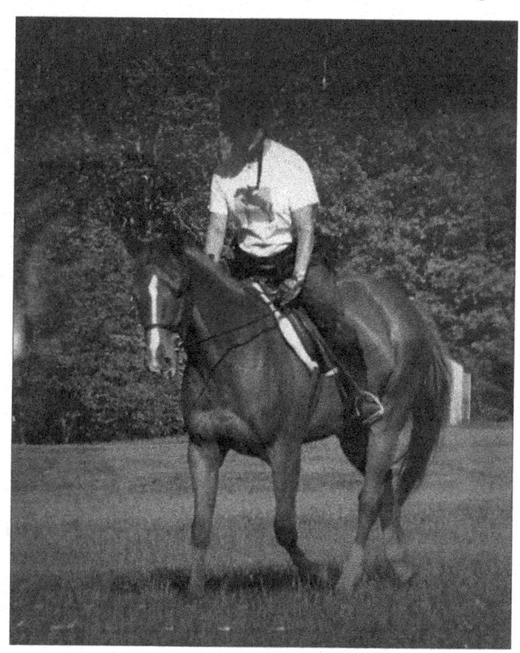

*Milwaukee Wolf*

After a few days in the round pen, I put him in a larger pasture by himself. He proceeded to run a great deal more than I wanted. I had twice called the vet at the track hoping to get some first-hand history on the tendon, but I was only able to speak to the vet's wife. She said her husband worked constantly, 7 days a week, and he never called me back. We increased Wolf 's turnout time, and he continued to run and trot in our pastures with his tail over his back—absolutely sound! The summer flies bothered him, and he started to lose weight despite the excellent summer pasture, so we increased his grain.

We had good rains through June and July, and our pastures were soft and lush when he arrived. On July 25th, Wolf was left in his stall 14 hours waiting for the rain to stop, and he came out of his stall really sore footed. I checked his digital pulse, and he had an easily detectable pulse in both front feet. He had actually lost weight his first eight days on our farm, due to the turnout time and the summer flies and mosquitoes. He was still most likely being fed considerably less grain than a week earlier at the track, but I didn't know for sure because I never met the trainer, and my Spanish is not good enough to have had a meaningful conversation with either his groom or the barn foreman. There was absolutely no doubt that the sore feet coming out of the stall on July 25th was acute laminitis, but I did not treat him with any Bute because he was walking fine by the time he got out of the barn, and he took off running sound again as soon as he was turned loose in the pasture. I did reduce his grain slightly because I felt he was on the verge of more serious laminitis. He got thinner than I liked over the next couple months as I tried to balance how much excellent pasture and grain his feet could tolerate.

The good rains stopped the last week of July, and our pastures quickly dried up and hardened. The grass lost its lushness with just a couple weeks of dry August heat. The farrier at the racetrack had removed his shoes the day before we picked him up. The first 14 days, while he was on the soft pasture, or in a stall, his feet looked very good. But now his thin hoof walls very quickly broke away on the hard ground, and he was walking on his soles by the second week of August. The running and playing suddenly stopped, as he quickly got very sore footed. Because I did not think his July 25th bout of acute laminitis was due to excessive grain, I was again increasing his grain and alfalfa to try to keep some weight on his bones.

From August 16 to 18, Wolf had a brief bout of acute laminitis with increased digital pulse strength which normalized after a couple doses of Bute and another temporary grain reduction. When he was over that three-day flare up, I had a farrier put firm rim casts on his front feet to protect what was left of his very thin hoof walls. He did not need more horseshoe nails in his very thin walls at that point. I already had him on Farrier's Formula 2X, but even with that great supplement, it would take about six weeks to get enough good hoof wall to grow down to where it could help the horse get the weight off his soles.

I had to trim out some of the rim casts a couple times, because they seemed to be putting too much pressure on certain spots of his soles. Just as we were about to go visit our son in Colorado for three days over Labor Day weekend, Wolf, who had been sore footed for most of a month, looked like he might be developing an abscess. I had to decide that afternoon whether to take the rim cast off after less than ten days, and search for an abscess, which would mean more work for our neighbor/horse sitter or leave some Bute if he got more sore while we were gone. I guessed wrong, and we returned home after the holiday weekend to a very sore footed horse with an obvious abscess.

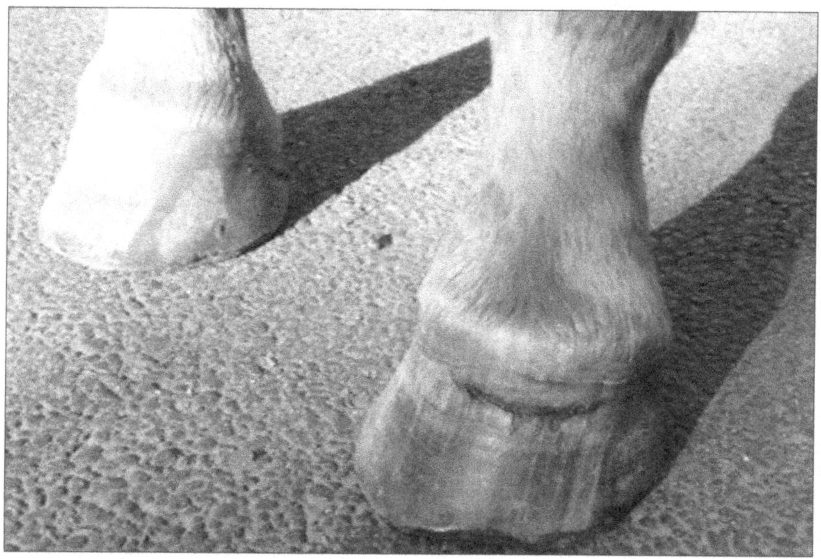

*Milwaukee Wolf's Hoof Abscess*

I took the casts off, opened the abscess at the toe, and wrapped his foot with a diaper and heavy duct tape over iodine and Epsom salts. Usually, my diaper and duct tape will easily last two or three days before it needs to be changed, but because the ground was still so hard, I was lucky when it lasted two days, more often having to change it every day. While he was healing from the abscess, I observed a third, and more significant, attack of acute laminitis from September 16 to 18. I had to reduce his grain and alfalfa again, reduce his stall time, and give him a couple more doses of Bute before the digital pulse stayed normal again after three days. While these three bouts of mild acute laminitis were going on, Wolf never stood rocked back on his heels, but it was very easy to see his lameness if we left him in the stall too long. Turning him out quickly softened his digital pulse, with or without Bute, as he walked around the dry paddock or the grass pastures.

I compare this to me sitting on an airplane, or in a movie theater too long, with tight shoes on. No one but I will know that my feet are starting to hurt from lack of fresh blood flow. If I walk a couple minutes, my feet feel fine again. Sometimes the horse in the stall does not get taken out for a walk, so his feet keep hurting for 24 hours or more.

Wolf had been shod constantly since he was 2 years old, except for his 3-year-old year on the turnout farm, where he was in a paddock just five hours every day, and a very nicely bedded large stall the other 19 hours each day. Racehorses are shod as differently as human athletes. Whether a human is going dancing, playing soccer or basketball, digging ditches, or waitressing, the choice of shoes is very important. At the racetrack, the emphasis is on speed, so horses are generally shod with a very light shoe, and the hoof is generally not allowed to spread and get too big. Farriers call a thick hoof wall "flare," and most are constantly rasping it away. Horses run faster with a lighter, smaller foot, than with the big round foot we like to see on trail horses. With the constant resets and new shoeings at the track, Wolf 's hooves had always been rasped rather thin. Now that he was on our farm, in dry, hard August paddocks, he needed the protection of much stronger hoof sidewalls.

It was a very difficult balancing act trying to keep the weight on his bones in fly season while fighting persistent, recurring mild acute laminitis caused by the hard ground and lack of hoof wall. The three-day delay in opening the abscess at the toe caused some of the abscess to travel up the front of the hoof wall and open at the coronary band a week later. This later proved to be a very significant timeline marker, as a significant size hole and fever ring grew down the hoof wall over the next eight months. In addition to the definite fever ring

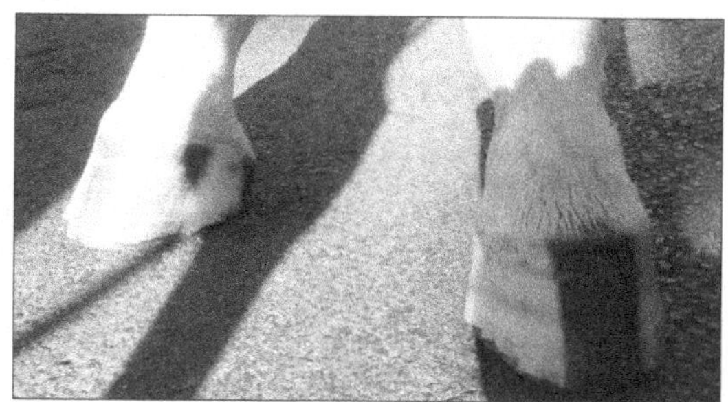

*Milwaukee Wolf's Hoof Rings*

from the abscess and inflammation the last week of August and first week of September, there was also a previous ring growing down about 5/8 inch lower—on all 4 hooves! The upper ring aligned with the abscess hole also was on all four feet, and actually more easily seen on Wolf 's hind feet, which are white striped. The lower ring was from his last month at the track when the trainer and vet decided he needed a year off for a tendon which turned out to be not at all sore. He ran hard and fast in the pasture, with no tenderness, when he first arrived on our farm.

These two separate fever rings on all four feet were the proof, months after the fact, that Wolf had persistent low-grade laminitis in all four feet in June, about a month before we picked him up, and again in August, a month after we brought him home. I had only seen it on five of those days, but the width of the two visible growth rings from all four coronary bands told me it was more persistent than just five days. Without seeing Wolf walk out of his stall after standing for several hours, most vets would never have suspected this horse might have acute laminitis at the racetrack or on our farm. They now call this "subclinical laminitis," or "too mild to detect," but it can cause damage unnoticed.

At any racetrack, you see horses constantly being walked in the shed rows. The trainers may not suspect laminitis, but they know walking is far better for a horse's circulation than standing in a stall. This is exactly why nearly all orthopedic surgeons make their patients get out of bed and walk the hospital aisles a day after replacing their hip or knee. MDs know patients heal better with better circulation, and you simply do not get optimum circulation to your feet or legs lying in bed or standing in a stall!

In my opinion, standing in stalls too long, and insufficient Bute, are the two biggest reasons why, according to multiple reports, 50% of horses who develop laminitis in hospitals are eventually euthanized. Acute laminitis must be recognized early, and treated properly, during the window of opportunity to prevent foundering your horse. Any living tissue deprived of fresh oxygen, by a less than optimum blood supply, will start to degenerate and die. You must recognize acute laminitis and immediately start to reduce the laminar swelling and edema of inflammation to prevent laminar damage. Cold water hosing and gentle walking on soft ground with properly trimmed feet, can be extremely effective in preventing laminar damage when acute laminitis, no matter how mild or severe, is recognized early.

We took Wolf and Breeze to the Carolina foothills on a three-week vacation from January to February 2014. Bill O'Neill, one of the very finest journeymen farriers, trimmed him. From his feet being painfully short and sore in August and September 2013, Bill said they were textbook perfect by the following February. I had been feeding him Farrier's Formula 2X for six months by then, and the August drought had been followed by good rains and early snow. I had only lightly shaped his hooves with a rasp the prior six months.

The next two summers, 2014 and 2015, Wolf had several more very minor bouts of mild acute laminitis. Because of his metabolism, he always required much more grain and good hay to look fit. He had never been fat. Sometimes when the grass is lush, or he is left in his stall too long after eating, he will come out a little tender footed. I can feel a digital pulse, which will disappear after five minutes in the pasture or round pen. His feet now have far thicker walls and soles due to Farriers Formula 2X, and no horseshoe nails! He is not in any danger of founder as long as someone knows how to recognize and treat acute laminitis.

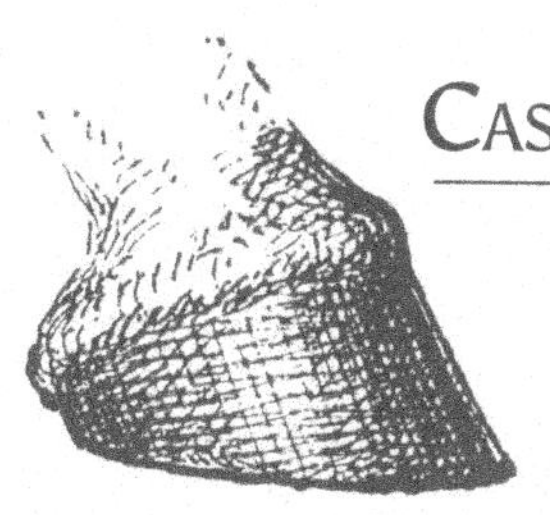

## Case Study

# "Warm Breeze"

### *Diagnosing Acute Laminitis, Even When You Cannot See Lameness*

ON MONDAY MORNING, MAY 21, 2012, my wife Julie rode to our back door and started hollering for me to come out and check her horse. She was sitting on Warm Breeze, her new Palomino gelding who was still two weeks short of his third birthday. She was very upset that he was "not right" and wanted an immediate answer. She told me he had been lying down in his stall after his small breakfast of a half can of grain. She was very pleased that he let her trim his bridle path while he was still lying down, a good display of confidence in a young horse. He was perfect when she saddled him and rode him back to the arena at a walk, but when she asked him to trot, he was just "not right." She thought he might have laminitis. We had been out of town for three days and I did not know how much pasture, alfalfa, or grain he had received the past three days. Our son, who had been feeding him over the weekend, was already off to school that morning. I reached down and could not feel a digital pulse behind either front fetlock. I needed to see Breeze trot on the black top road in front of our house, so Julie rode down the driveway to the road. If it was laminitis, I expected he would be worse if I held up one foot for 30 seconds.

I asked Julie to trot off after holding up Breeze's right front foot for half a minute. I did not see him favor the left front leg, but she immediately returned and declared it was "much worse." I told her it was very mild laminitis, although I did not see it. I gave him 5 cc (1 gram) of Bute IV with her still in the saddle. I told her to take him on a long walk, and he should be better in 10 minutes.

While she was gone, I remembered that we had stuffed a nearly full bale of alfalfa into a hay net and hung it in his lean-to on Thursday night before we left town. We expected him to be left with 31-year-old Casey in a large paddock with short grass and a lean-to while we were out of town, and our teenage son was very busy in school all day. Breeze was normally kind to old Casey, but apparently Breeze didn't share his hanging bale of alfalfa.

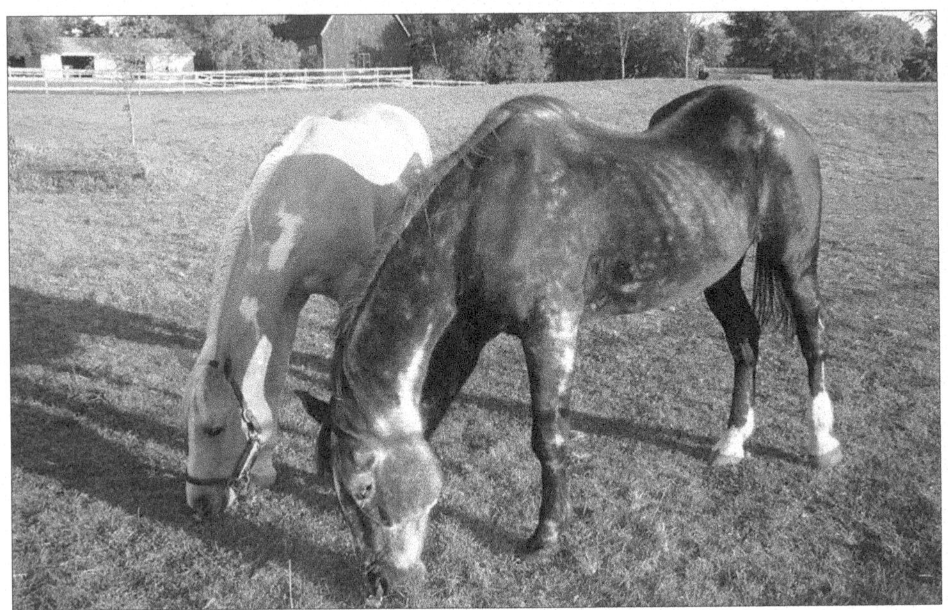

*Warm Breeze and Casey*

When Julie came back from her 40-minute walk, Breeze was better, but still "not quite right" when she had asked him to trot in the grass arena. We put him in the paddock with the short grass all day, and she rode him again that evening. She said he was then much better, but still she rode him very lightly. The next day he was "outstanding," her term for good progress.

By Wednesday, after a full riding session he was listening, working, and moving the best since she had bought him the previous October. She had gone from a very upset wife to a very happy wife in just 48 hours with a single injection of 5 cc (1gm) of Bute and correcting our feeding mistake. If we had not cut back his alfalfa, grain, and good grass, or if we had left him in a stall, or if he had been shod, his recovery would not have been quite so fast and complete. Recovery also would have taken longer if Breeze had been overweight.

Of the five horses in which I have caused a total of 15 episodes of laminitis the past 42 years, none were fat, and all were fully recovered within a week. Unfortunately, most riders do not think of laminitis when they first feel their horse is slightly off. This allows the very mild acute laminitis to linger for days, or sometimes weeks, before it is diagnosed and corrected. If identified early by both a sensitive rider and a vet who can diagnose it without needing to see bone X-rays, acute laminitis should be fully curable with zero permanent damage.

Four years later, the now 7-year-old Breeze had moved to South Carolina with us. His last three years in Illinois he has had five brief and mild acute laminitis attacks. My wife is an international flight attendant and is typically out of town for three days about three or four times a month. If Breeze has an attack when Julie is out of town, it will leave a growth ring on his hoof that shows up a month later and grows to the ground in eight or ten months. If Julie is in town, she will discover it the first day, and we can immediately cut back on pasture, alfalfa, grain, or stall time with no hoof damage.

Researchers now call this "subclinical laminitis," but it is very real and will get worse if not recognized and treated. It can be detected by a good rider, and it can be demonstrated with a good exam.

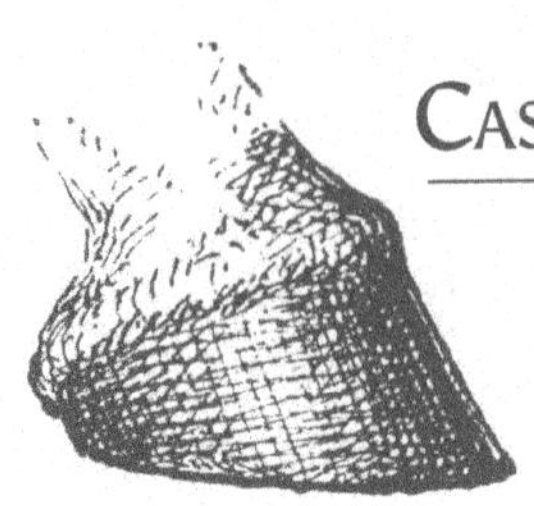

# Case Study

## "Dom Perignon"

### *Very Brief and Fatal*

I ONLY KNEW DOM PERIGNON for a week, but I will never forget his story because he was one of just two horses I have had to euthanize for laminitis. Dom was an off the track Thoroughbred in his late teens at a hunter/jumper show stable which I had only previously visited a couple times for pre-purchase exams, and one emergency colic. The vast majority of the horses in jumping stables like this are privately owned, but they are usually under the daily care and management of a professional trainer. Some owners see their horse almost every day while others may only get to the barn a few times a month. Typically, the professional trainer arranges all the veterinary care.

When I was first called by Judy, Dom's vary caring owner, he was not overweight, and he was shod with full pads. Judy told me Dom had been diagnosed with laminitis three weeks earlier. He had been given a variety of medications including Bute, acepromazine and heparin. But his laminitis progressed, despite everything the regular vet advised. He had been taken off Bute despite his severe pain because "Bute could cause ulcers." He was still being fed a rich alfalfa hay and a moderate amount of grain twice a day. The horse was in his stall in severe pain with Grade IV laminitis, confined there because they were afraid it was too dangerous to let him walk. The X-rays showed dramatically worsening rotation over just three weeks' time. Now the vet and trainer were advising the owner to put Dom to sleep, because nothing they tried had helped him.

Judy listened carefully to my treatment protocol, which I told her is best used much earlier in the disease. We did not have the option to roll back the clock, so we put Dom back on Bute, removed his shoes, trimmed his toes and heels a little, and turned him out in the indoor arena overnight, with the trainer's permission. We put a flake of hay, with the alfalfa leaves shaken out, in each of the four corners. Dom wandered the arena all night.

Judy called the next morning to say that he was walking better than he had in nearly a month. I advised her to reduce the Bute dosage and continue as much indoor arena time as possible. The other horses needed to work in the arena during the day and early evening, so I do not know how long Dom stayed in his stall each day.

I rechecked Dom with Judy three days later which unfortunately was about the 30th day for Dom's laminitis. He was indeed walking much better. The Bute had been reduced to just 1 gram twice a day. I trimmed some more toe off his still too long feet and lowered his heels more to get his frog closer to the ground. She reported that he did very well for two more days. On Saturday morning, he could not get up in his stall.

My wife had invited nearly 100 friends and clients for my 50th birthday party, when I received Judy's desperate Saturday morning call. When I arrived, it was evident that Dom's coffin bones had penetrated both front soles in his stall overnight, and there was no reason to prolong his pain with this complication. I euthanized him, but I still remember his brief case from 23 years ago like it was yesterday. The three weeks of inappropriate drugs and stall confinement without removing his shoes severely damaged his feet. Then, trying to walk a horse with severe laminitis at that stage was obviously too little, too late.

If you contrast this case with so many of the other stories in this book (Spirit, Dots, Cody, Bradley, Dixie, etc.), each was more severe and acute in onset, but all were diagnosed and treated correctly from day one. For every failure like Dom, I have 50 successes that returned to their full prior use. Luck and the "mysterious nature of the disease" have nothing to do with it. The 45 years and hundreds of research articles published on laminitis since I started vet school have not changed my inflammation and vasocompression theory, or my basic treatment of laminitis. The research in most all cases has been consistent with what I have believed all along. The researchers and professors who try to make the research fit their basic vasoconstriction theory remain mystified. It is the hospital doctors who see the horses too late, and without the benefit of sand arenas for 24-hour turnout, who remain most frustrated of all. Laminitis seen early is the easiest disease I get to treat; if seen too late, it is the worst.

# ~SECTION XII~

## Inappropriate Conditions

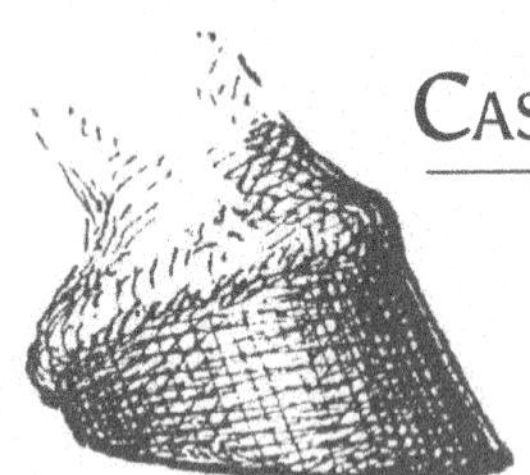

## Case Study

# "Painter"

*They said, "He was never lame."*

THIS IS ONE OF MY most difficult stories, and the most heavily disguised, because of the people involved. All the names and dates have been changed, but what happened to this horse is painfully true.

Kristi was one of my favorite clients, who took outstanding care of her three horses on her small farm. I became her veterinarian 15 years earlier after she received a very poor prognosis, and very expensive treatment plan, from her vet for laminitis in one of her mares. After switching vets, her mare did beautifully, and she gave me all the credit. It was a simple case, with a very quick and full recovery. It was much less significant to me than to her because it was so typical of what I had seen hundreds of times the prior 20 years.

Despite really good personal care of her three horses, Kristi unbelievably lost two very healthy mares to colic. She called me quickly in both cases, and they were quickly referred to an outstanding hospital just 15 miles away, where both died, about a year apart, despite the surgeon's best efforts.

Kristi replaced these two very nice mares with Painter's mother when she was a green broke 3-year-old in foal with Painter. The home foaling was difficult, he did not nurse well, and required IgG hyperimmune plasma and intensive care from Kristi the first week of his life. Painter survived and grew into a large, powerful, and very spoiled paint horse.

Painter was barely green-broke when he rolled into a fence as a 3-year-old. He injured a rear hoof so badly, we referred him to a hospital where the surgeon showed Kristi a fractured rear coffin bone with a hoof injury which would require removal of about 1/3 of the lateral hoof wall. The surgeon advised a screw for the coffin bone. I advised Kristi to have the hospital's expert farrier resect the hoof wall, apply a bar shoe, and bring the horse home. This was just a year after Barbaro had been in the news for his opposite hoof laminitis after his right hind leg fractures, and the surgeon was worried it might occur in Painter. I knew that at home Painter would not be locked in a hospital stall for six weeks. The bar shoe and the remaining hoof wall would serve as a cast, and Painter would rest the hoof because he would not be on the level of pain killers which allowed Barbaro to scratch his left ear with his left hind foot two days after surgery on the right hind leg.

Kristi took care of Painter's injury herself and brought him back to the hospital every third or fourth week to have the bar shoe reset, and his coffin bone was healed by the eighth week. The hoof took over six months to grow out, but Painter was quite sound by the sixth week. He did miss most of his planned training as a 3-year-old.

In the spring as a 4-year-old, Painter was way too much horse for Kristi to train herself, so she sent him to a farm where there was a very arrogant trainer. He had called me the past three years only to draw Coggins tests on the eight to ten horses in his barn. He never asked me for any other veterinary care. The third year, I noticed that one of his mares was badly foundered. She had been normal the year before, but was now shod, with obviously damaged feet. I asked him what happened. His reply was, "She foundered. I did everything I could for her" (except call a vet). "There's nothing else they could have done," he said.

I was not happy Painter had gone there and told Kristi exactly that. Nevertheless, he stayed there until he also foundered, without ever showing the know-it-all trainer any lameness. I got to see Painter weeks after the damage was done. He was trail sound, but he had very unnecessary damage to his feet. It would never have happened if the arrogant trainer had not so intimidated the wonderful owner. Not everyone is the expert they think they are, and many do not know what they don't know.

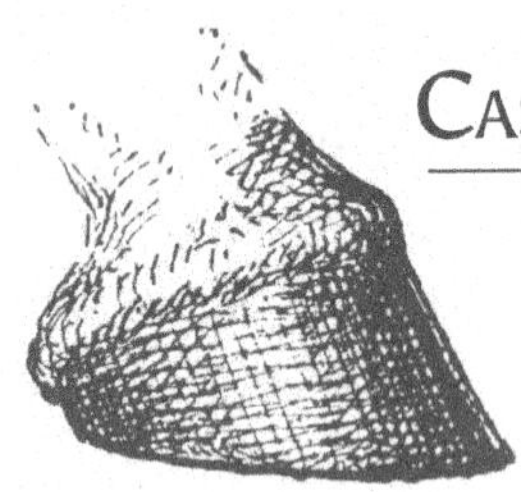

## Case Study

# "Omar"

### *Foundered By Five Bad Human Errors*

OMAR IS A CLASSIC EXAMPLE OF a horse who foundered unnoticed by his owner, a vet clinic barn manager, a farrier, and two vets in the acute stage. Omar was a 10-year-old Arabian gelding who moved from out of state with his owner Kim, and her six other horses, to a brand new 5-acre horse farm about ten minutes from my farm. Kim was a well-educated horse owner. A prior out-of-state vet had "diagnosed the blood clot" two years earlier and treated Omar twice with two 5-day courses of chelation therapy. The first year and a half of our veterinarian-client-patient relationship everyone was very happy. Then Kim announced in late February 1989 that Omar was "off" again, and she was sure it was a blood clot in one of his iliac arteries leading to a rear leg. Kim felt the chelation therapy had helped him, and she wanted me to do it for him again. She did let me do a rectal exam first, and I felt identical, normal pulse pressures in all four iliac arteries. I did not have an ultrasound machine in 1989 to further search for any evidence of arterial obstruction.

I had no training in chelation therapy and had never been asked to administer it before, or since. I had learned from my years with harness racing horses that if a trainer believes they need a treatment, you sometimes do have to accommodate them or they will simply find another vet who will give them what they want.

I was asked to call the out of state vet, who gave me his formula for a variety of vitamins, minerals, EDTA, and other drugs to be diluted in a liter of 5% dextrose and given by slow IV drip over 45 minutes for five days in a row. Since the weather was still very cold and rainy, and the procedure so long for 5 days in a row, I requested that the horse be boarded at a nearby equine clinic if I was to do this, which I did not believe was necessary for the horse.

Normally, a liter of IV fluids, which are commonly given to restore electrolytes at the racetrack, takes about ten minutes. Standing beside a horse, holding a jug of fluids for 45 minutes required more patience than I had. After about 15 minutes the first day, I handed the chelation fluids to the clinic manager. I was assured that they could complete the infusion without me watching, and I left for my other calls. I drove to the clinic and started the IV solution five days in a row, then left with instructions that they were supposed to regulate the speed of the infusion by raising or lowering the fluids so that gravity would slow the administration as needed to finish in about 45 minutes.

I did not hear from Kim again until June 17, when she called me out for spring booster vaccinations. When Kim brought Omar out of his stall, the very first thing I saw was a really large fever ring about 1 to 1¼ inches below each coronary band. Incredibly, Kim had not noticed the rings before I pointed them out. I asked her what had happened in the three months since I had last seen Omar. She said the chelation did not seem to help him as much as in the prior years, and that she had been giving him 2 grams of Bute most days to keep him more comfortable.

He was in a stall every night and fed grain and good alfalfa hay day and night. He had limited pasture, but it had gone through the normal northern Illinois spring flush of rapid growth. All the while he had laminitis, but Kim never suspected it. His white line was widely separated, and his soles were seriously dropped. His farrier had trimmed the horse a few weeks earlier but had not mentioned anything to Kim. Possibly the horse was new to him, and he thought this was normal for this horse. I X-rayed Omar that day and he was rotated 12 degrees, fully foundered.

I trimmed Omar myself several times the next sixty days. By rasping back his front hoof walls the angle of rotation was reduced, but the damage was done to his laminae. I spoke with the clinic vet who had seen Omar in his barn for five days. The barn manager then told me that each day about an hour after each infusion Omar had broken out into a heavy sweat. This was a very common reaction to a commonly used hormone to induce ovulation on breeding farms at the time, so the barn manager did not think it was significant enough to mention to me when I came to start the next infusion each day.

Kim switched vets that fall, and within three years Omar reportedly had more serious relapses of laminitis that were treated with stall rest, therapeutic shoes, and vasodilating drugs, but which left him permanently lame.

If you have lost track of all the errors in killing Omar, the worst were:

1. He probably never had an iliac thrombosis, but the prior vet told the owner something she thought helped her horse.
2. I was willing to give the horse something I did not believe he needed in order to not lose a client.
3. I did not do a lameness exam. I only checked for an iliac thrombosis, found none and treated the horse anyway for the owner.
4. The barn manager failed to mention an unexpected side effect.
5. The clinic vet also failed to tell me about the side effect of the infusions.
6. Kim treated the horse for three months with Bute without telling her vet.
7. The shoer did not mention to Kim that her horse was foundered.

Yes, Dr. MacKay-Smith, some horses can founder without someone noticing, but do not tell me no one did anything wrong! It is only by naming and claiming our mistakes that we can hope to prevent them next time.

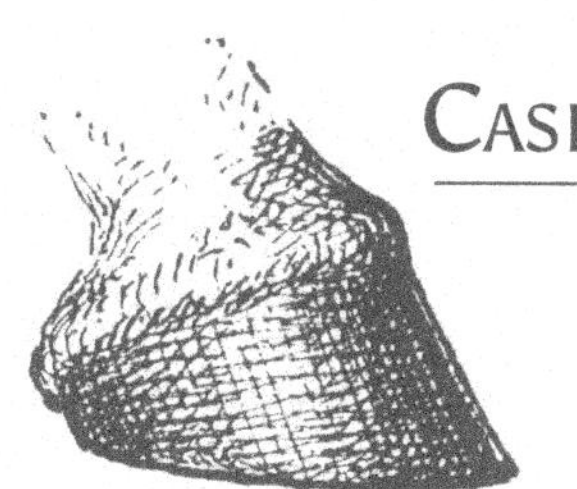

## Case Study

# "Jana" and "Flash"

### *Two Veterinarians Misdiagnosed Acute Laminitis from Summer Clover Within a Month*

JANA AND FLASH ARE TWO VERY different horses with long and different histories, who had very similar misdiagnosed cases of pasture laminitis in the summer of 2010. At least three times I have seen nationally prominent veterinarians write in prestigious publications that sometimes laminitis skips the acute stage. They sincerely believe that sometimes a horse which was extremely well cared for on a daily basis just shows up with rotated coffin bones on the first day of lameness and nobody missed anything. Researchers also write that by the time a horse with acute laminitis shows lameness, there is already permanent damage to his laminae.

By 2015, academic vets, researchers, and professors started calling these cases "subclinical laminitis." Apparently, that is because they cannot diagnose it with current technology.

I have always considered these mild cases the most dangerous because they are harder to diagnose. The vet has to suspect it might be laminitis, then confirm or exclude it with a careful physical exam. Radiographs are not useful and can only show that a coffin bone has moved after the fact. A horse will have acute laminitis before there is movement of the coffin bone. "Subclinical laminitis" makes as much sense to me as subclinical pregnancy or subclinical cancer. Just because the diagnosis was delayed does not mean the pregnancy, the cancer or the laminitis skipped the acute stage.

Jana and Flash were misdiagnosed by excellent and very experienced equine practitioners. Drs. Smith and Jones (not partners, and not their real names) have very good reputations, with ten and forty years of private practice experience as exclusively equine practitioners. Neither has had a single malpractice suit of which I am aware. They both have the latest digital X-ray equipment, but they simply missed the diagnosis on these two horses in the mild acute stage when the owners called them last summer. It is politically incorrect, and some say unethical, to criticize another veterinarian, but horses will continue to suffer and die from uncontrollable founder unless someone points out their errors, which we all make as we "practice."

I was called to offer a second opinion for persistent lameness in both these cases. Jana and Flash are very different horses, and their eventual treatment and outcomes could not be more different, although the original cause of their laminitis was nearly identical.

Jana was a 13-year-old AQHA mare who had been a patient of mine for four years. She was a very solid mare with excellent, tough, round, black, well-shaped, barefoot hooves. She was one of four horses owned by Vicki and her two school- age daughters. Vicki was a regular client about ten or twelve years and always boarded her horses at various stables. As her daughters entered high school, she bought more horses for them to share, and she moved her horses to a farm where Jana was kept in a large pasture 24/7 with ten to fifteen other horses. All were well fed and Jana, being a dominant mare, always got a little more than her fair share of the grain dumped in the long manger twice a day by the hired farm workers. The horses were rotated on pastures that were sometimes rather lush, and other times pretty sparse, but always supplemented with good round bales. For four years Jana thrived in this situation and never had an injury or lameness of any sort. Her weight always looked very normal for her breed and type when I saw her for semi-annual vaccinations.

Vicki, the owner, died very suddenly and tragically in the spring of 2010. Her daughters, still in high school, sold two of their four horses, and Donna, one of the new buyers, called me for a copy of Jana's Coggins test. I was unaware that in June 2010 Jana started showing periodic shifting soreness. As a first-time horse owner, Donna called Dr. Jones, her riding partner's veterinarian, to check Jana's legs. Dr. Jones was not familiar with the 13-year-old mare, and seeing extremely little consistent soreness, he attributed what Donna saw to natural "age related arthritis." He prescribed minimal Bute as needed for trail riding. Donna continued to ride Jana all summer with occasional use of a gram or two of Bute.

Dr. Jones was asked to look at Jana a second time, later in the summer for the lingering mild "lameness." He again attributed it to "mild generalized arthritis." When the "arthritis" had persisted for about three months, Donna called me to administer her fall booster vaccination and offer another opinion about the new on and off "arthritis."

When I arrived, Donna was grooming Jana while tied to a post in the large pasture run in shed. As I vaccinated her, I told Donna I had never seen the mare so fat. She was always an easy keeper, but she now appeared to be about 60 to 80 pounds overweight. I ran my hands down her forelegs and found her fetlocks and pasterns very clean. Except for her weight she looked no different than I had seen her the past four years.

After the vaccination I sat down and discussed Jana's weight with Donna. I was trying to convince Donna that Jana needed to be separated from the herd at feeding time, because she was obviously getting far more grain than she needed, but this was going to be a nuisance for the farm workers. I was explaining the serious risk of laminitis to her, which was new to her, when I noticed Jana would shift her weight from side to side every 15 or 20 seconds. She would also occasionally lift a front foot momentarily while standing quietly tied to the post.

After at least ten minutes talking to Donna and watching her horse shift her weight unnaturally, it occurred to me that she might already have the laminitis I was describing. Being tied to a post in the aisle for 20 or 30 minutes slowed the circulation enough to make her uncomfortable. I was able to easily feel a moderate digital pulse at the base of her front fetlocks. Donna also felt the pulse, but we could not find a pulse in her hind fetlocks. I tapped on Jana's front hoof walls with my hoof testers. She immediately lifted her front feet off the ground. She ignored the same tapping on her rear feet. We then took her outside the barn, and she trotted normally away from me. She had no pain at all on flexion, but when I picked up her left front leg for 30 seconds, she trotted off lame on her right foot. I then repeated this test on the right side, and she trotted lame on the left front foot. I did not X-ray her because it would not have changed my diagnosis or treatment. In fact, the most likely thing an X-ray would have shown is no laminitis!

Thankfully, Jana had not been in a stall all summer, and her constant walking in the pasture had kept enough blood flowing to keep her laminae strong enough to not fail through three months of misdiagnosed acute laminitis. Six years later, the university experts began calling this "subclinical" laminitis. The occasional Bute for the supposed arthritis and the constant walking from the flies was enough treatment to prevent rotation despite three months of excessive clover, good pasture, and more than her fair share of grain.

That night, I sent Donna a half dozen of these laminitis stories. She took away Jana's grain while the pasture and clover were in bloom, and Jana's "arthritis" was cured. I only saw her a few more times. She lost weight quickly and did not have another problem of which I was aware.

Flash was a 19-year-old retired champion racehorse. His misdiagnosed acute laminitis happened at the same time, 30 miles away with a different vet, but on almost identical pasture and clover. His owner was told he was "sore footed" from stomping flies. Expensive digital X-rays showed he had no rotation. He was prescribed shoes, but no feed changes. He was stalled and pampered every night, and when I was called for a second opinion three weeks later, he was far down the road to founder. A year of very hard work was unable to save a wonderful horse.

Because of the difference in hoof quality, and every night in a stall, Flash had a far shorter window of opportunity to prevent fatal founder by correctly diagnosing and treating acute laminitis.

The reasons for success and failure in these two horses' bouts of laminitis had nothing to do with luck or the mysterious nature of the disease. They were totally due to the care they received before the damage was done. Staying out all night was what gave Jana a much longer window of opportunity for correct diagnosis and treatment. Do not accept the excuse that these two horses had "subclinical" laminitis. Both owners saw the lameness and called two very well qualified vets who simply missed the correct diagnosis.

# ~SECTION XIII~

## SHETLAND PONIES

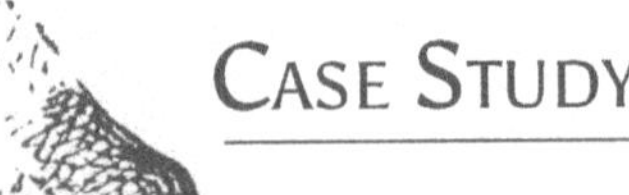

## Case Study

# "Elvis"

*14 Extra Good Years for a "Special Needs" Pony*

SINCE OPENING MY MOSTLY BACKYARD equine practice in the NW Chicago suburbs in 1974, there has been a shift in the type of horses kept by many of my clients. Whereas in the 1970s and '80s there were many clients breeding Arabs, Paints, Appaloosas, Warm Blood crosses, etc., and raising them on suburban 5-acre farms, by 2010 the backyard breeder had all but become extinct in my area. There were simply too many unwanted horses available for free. Nobody likes to euthanize a horse they no longer want to keep.

Elvis was an unbroken, short, prematurely arthritic, shaggy, and already foundered, 6-year-old Shetland pony when he was rescued from a pathological collector of a wide variety of neglected farm animals in 2001. He also was blind in one eye.

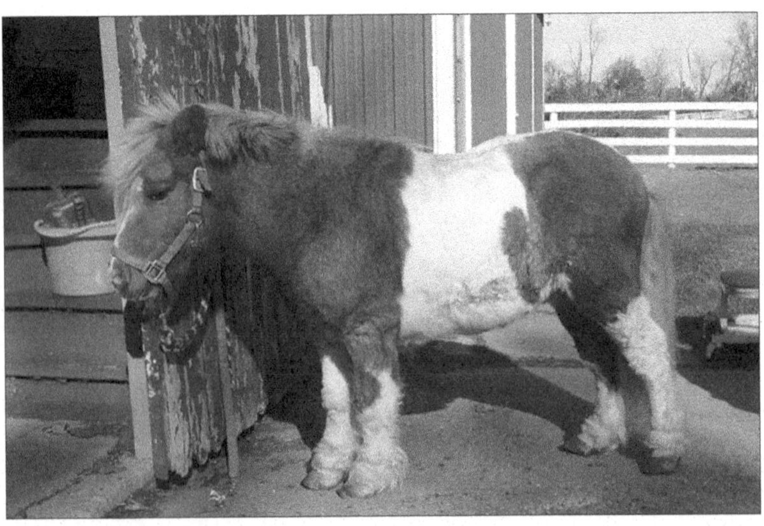

Elvis had been adopted by Jackie, an extremely kind, dedicated, intelligent, and reasonable animal lover, because no one else would take him. His feet were badly overgrown, and he was very difficult to trim due to his lack of prior handling, soreness, poor lateral flexibility, and very short legs. The first farrier insisted on trimming him holding a foot between his legs. This pulled the leg sideways out from under the pony, and he had to be tranquilized for trimming. When it became too difficult to coordinate my visits with this farrier, I simply trimmed Elvis myself, not pulling his leg so far laterally. Jackie finally found another farrier who was equally patient with Elvis' limited flexibility.

Jackie usually fed a little bit too much, and she had to keep the pony in a stall every night, but she had prior experience with foundered ponies and a very big heart. She also had a large pasture where Elvis was allowed to roam and graze just a few hours a day when it was not too lush. He would then come into a dry lot and his softly bedded box stall that he often shared with a goat at night. More on that goat's digestive system causing some of Elvis' suffering in his final days follows below.

Elvis had only three moderate and easily resolved laminitis flare ups his first four years with Jackie. His first flare-up was on August 23, 2002. While the pasture looked pretty safe for Elvis because it was a hot, dry summer, there were some areas of very short clover which the little pony was able to graze closer than the horses because of his thin lips. This was before grazing muzzles became popular to limit grazing on pasture. His second flare up was a year and a half later, February 24, 2004, after eating grass hay that had gone to seed. August 24, 2005, he had a third episode, again blamed on very short clover in the pasture which he could eat closer than the horses. Each of the first three laminitis relapses responded nicely to just a couple weeks of progressively lower doses of Bute, and removal from the pasture or shaking out the hay.

On May 10, 2006, five years after adoption, he had his first major flare up from very rapidly growing spring pasture. This was before I understood the connection between plant sugars or Non-Structural Carbohydrates (NSCs) and laminitis. When pasture is growing very fast due to the right combination of temperature, rain, and sunshine, photosynthesis makes more sugars (simple carbohydrates) than the plant can use for growth during the daylight hours. The grass can grow an inch overnight as it converts the NSCs to plant fiber. We always called this lush pasture, which apparently is not as great a problem in other areas of the country. During rapid growing seasons, the pasture is safer in the morning, than in the afternoon as the NSCs can build up quickly during the day.

From 2007 to 2015, Elvis had a flare up every August no matter how careful Jackie was with the pasture and muzzles. It always took about two months to get him through his annual August to September flare ups. The other ten months of each year he was Bute free and pasture sound. Jackie would often just come over to pick up another 50 grams of Bute powder. She was the one who decided each day how sore he was and how much he needed. My instructions were always the minimum effective daily dose, not to exceed 2 grams. Often, her idea of how much he needed was a little higher than mine, but she kept him comfortable to her standards while I worried about the side effects of long-term Bute. Then he would be good for another ten months before the laminitis and Bute started up again.

After several years when we could not blame it on pasture, we began looking more carefully at the walnut trees that overhung his dry lot. He never ate the bark off these trees, nor were there shoots with any leaves eaten. The leaves usually started to fall in August and while we never saw him show any interest in even eating a fallen leaf, Jackie would rake the paddock leaves frequently. I believed in the end that Elvis had developed such a hypersensitivity to walnut leaves that just walking on them with his light-colored feet would set off his laminitis. I have never had a horse get laminitis from walnut stall shavings (40), but I do know of one large stable where about 30 of 300 horses got laminitis from a semi-trailer full of walnut shavings. Possibly light-colored feet absorb the allergen or toxin more easily, and perhaps Elvis was sensitized like some people are to peanuts or bee stings.

In 2014, Elvis developed a large abscess below his good eye that swelled enough to make him totally blind for a day until we got it drained. It was a foul-smelling mess that I attributed to a cheek ulcer in his mouth getting infected. It was hard to tell if the ulcer was from the Bute or his sharp molars. We did have the expensive dentist float him once with tiny instruments, because my horse-sized instruments were too big for his tiny mouth. Bob and Jackie diligently flushed the draining abscess a couple times a day for about three weeks, and the ugly wound healed without a trace of scar.

In 2015, the final blow for Elvis was a bizarre case of Wooden Tongue. This is a cattle disease that is never mentioned in equine medicine textbooks. Jackie found Elvis one morning gasping for breath with his tongue sticking out of his mouth. I was unable to get the tongue back in his mouth. It was stiff and swollen, longer and about double normal thickness, and his jaws were clamped on it like a horse with tetanus (lock jaw). I remembered hearing about Wooden Tongue 45 years earlier in vet school, but I had never seen a case. I put Elvis on a large tank of my personal oxygen supply and then called my cattle vet friend. He came over, confirmed the diagnosis, and administered sodium iodide, which quickly reduced the tongue swelling. Unfortunately, while Elvis was now able to get his tongue back in his mouth, he lost the full thickness mucosa from the front one inch of his tongue. With this new large and apparently painful ulcer, he simply refused to eat. He seemed very depressed and after three more days we decided he was telling us he had had enough.

The laminitis did not kill him, but one side effect of too much Bute is ulcers. Also, Elvis usually shared his stall with a goat. The Actinobacillus that causes Wooden Tongue disease is a normal inhabitant of a goat's ruminant, "bring it up to chew it again," digestive system. Elvis' feet were very well trimmed and almost normal looking for a pony who had so many flare ups of laminitis for so many years. The Bute may have been responsible for his eventual death, but it also gave him a lot of great days for 14 extra years. The story of Mary, the one other pony I had on daily Bute for over 20 years, is next. Although it is all too easy to overdose and kill a pony in a week with too much Bute, Elvis and Mary certainly benefited from prolonged use of minimal effective doses of this anti-inflammatory drug.

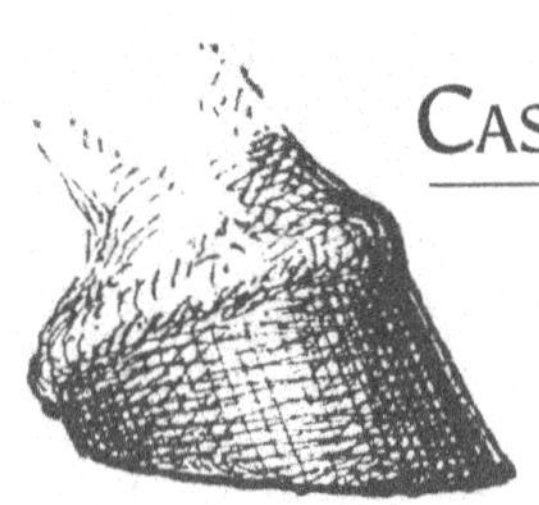

## Case Study

# "Mary" and "Frosty"

### *Daily Bute for 15 Years and 5 Years Respectively*

ONLY THE NAMES HAVE BEEN changed of this Shetland Pony mare and Quarter Horse mare to respect the privacy of two extremely dedicated clients. Many veterinarians will warn owners with horses in the initial stages of laminitis that if their horse is lucky enough to survive the initial attack, they are likely to permanently require expensive and difficult management. Some veterinarians specialize in treating these laminitis disasters, and on occasion they work miracles to salvage these cases for owners with unlimited resources. Eventual fatality rates for these extreme cases are about 90%.

I have had very limited experience with these types of cases because I have always focused on preventing complications by recognizing and correctly treating acute laminitis before it is too late. Of my more than 1,200 cases in 42 years, I only euthanized 26, and Mary and Frosty are the only two I remember who needed Bute every day for the rest of their lives. They were both kept barefoot but required more frequent expert trimming.

Mary, the Shetland pony, and Frosty, the Quarter Horse mare, each had an unusual owner who absolutely did not believe in euthanasia for horses that were just not sound enough to ride. Both owners believed if their horses were up, eating well, on whatever pain medication was necessary, and happy to see them, not being able to run and play was better than being dead. These two mares always had a great appetite and attitude, and neither horse ever had a single pressure sore from lying down too much.

Mary was a wonderfully trained younger Shetland Pony who was loaned by her longtime owner to various families throughout the 1970s as a mount for younger children to start the first season of Pony Club. About once a year during that time I had to treat Mary for a flare up of mild pasture laminitis. Each time she would be back to light work in a couple weeks with a short-term modest amount of Bute, some corrective trimming, and a diet and pasture lecture for the people using her that summer.

Mary's owner died in 1979, and another lady adopted Mary with the intention of continuing the annual summertime practice of loaning her to start another small child with horses. Mary would happily pop over tiny fences, and the smallest children didn't have too far to fall if they lost their seat. Unfortunately, Mary went along when her new owner was transferred to St. Louis for three years. When Mary returned, in the early 1980s, her laminitis was much worse and more difficult to treat, after the vasodilators, anticoagulants, stall rest, and less strict diet restrictions that she had received in the St. Louis area. At that time there was a great deal of laminitis research being done at the University of Missouri implicating endotoxemia as the primary cause of laminitis. Anti-endotoxin serums and even an endotoxemia/laminitis vaccine were released commercially with a heavy advertising campaign from the professor who developed them.

The vaccine sounded good in theory, so I bought 10 doses and tried the vaccine on Mary. From that day forward she was never sound enough to be ridden and was on constant daily Bute for about 15 more years. The vaccine disappeared from the market within the first year. Mary required and received excellent frequent trimming, as well as very careful diet and pasture supervision. I recommended she receive the minimum effective daily dose of ½ to 1 ½ grams of Bute per day for a pony her size. The property owners ignored my advice and gave her 1 to 3 grams every day for years and years. I was wary of the toxicity reported with Bute especially in ponies, and I repeatedly warned the owner and caretakers about Bute overdoses. Mary defied the research reports for about fifteen years. When Mary turned 30, she started developing huge bone spurs in her knees, most likely from the inhibition of articular cartilage regeneration from such long-term Bute use. It became very difficult for the farrier to bend her knees enough to trim her feet, but they managed to continue a few more years. Mary then had three separate colics within a year, most likely due to ulcers from the long-term Bute. Her owner finally allowed me to euthanize Mary during the third severe colic.

With the exception of her three years in St. Louis, I managed Mary's laminitis for 25 years and since she was already an experienced jumping Shetland when I met her, I estimate she was about 35 when she died. The very liberal use of Bute allowed her to live an additional 15 years.

I was first called to treat Frosty when her previous vet advised euthanasia for the 23-year-old AQHA mare due to severe founder. This was unacceptable to the owner, so she called me for a second opinion. According to the owner, Frosty had her first (of many) laminitis attacks at about the age of 5. The prior vet had treated her for founder many times the past 18 years, but he had enough. Her coffin bones were badly rotated, and he refused to continue prolonging such an uncomfortable life.

Incredibly, this mare was still being fed nearly pure alfalfa hay. No one had ever explained to this first-time horse owner that alfalfa and clover hays were as bad as grain and spring pasture for chronic laminitis. I immediately started Frosty on 4 grams of Bute per day. We switched her from the alfalfa hay to strictly grass hay. Most local horse hay grown in northern Illinois or southern Wisconsin has at least some alfalfa or clover mixed in the hay fields. Pure alfalfa hay is readily available, but better suited for dairy cattle. The relatively limited pure grass hay locally available is even sometimes too rich if it is cut after it has gone to seed. These later first cuttings containing seeds must also be avoided for laminitic horses.

With excellent daily care from her owner and an outstanding farrier, Frosty lived another five years at a different boarding stable. She was never able to run and play when turned out. She spent the vast majority of her time in a stall, and when I finally told the owner I also could no longer continue to participate in keeping Mary alive, I learned the farrier had told her the same thing on her last visit two weeks earlier.

The owner still was not ready to let Frosty be euthanized, but the next week Frosty developed very severe stress induced asthma that did not respond to any normal medications. I had to put Frosty to sleep because she could hardly breath. I have seen such stress induced asthma only four or five other times in 42 years treating thousands of horses.

Mary and Frosty demonstrate that not only is it easier to prevent than cure founder, but that the time for euthanasia is a very personal decision by the owner, and that horses with severe inflammation can tolerate maximum doses of Bute for much longer times than normal, healthy horses for whom one gram is an overdose.

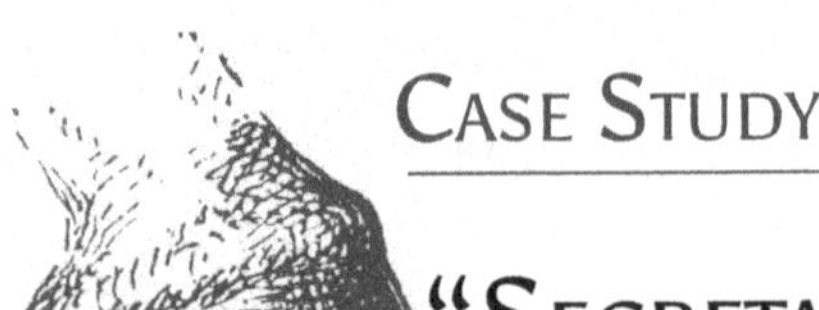

## Case Study

# "Secretariat" and "Snowman"

### *Very Little Public Information*

SECRETARIAT AND SNOWMAN WERE TWO more legendary horses who were euthanized due to "incurable" laminitis, while I was routinely curing the disease whenever I was called before rotation (and made the correct diagnosis). Both Secretariat's and Snowman's diseases were much more private than Barbaro's, but both horses had books published with accounts of their deaths. I also saw movies about both horses' lives and will make a few comments on their laminitis based strictly on what those books and movies have already put into the public record. Obviously, I would have loved to see either horse or discussed them with the treating veterinarians when I might have been able to help them. I have no idea who saw Secretariat, and Snowman's vet never returned my phone calls. Most vets simply do not like to talk about horses they lose, but it is usually after losses that I have learned the most.

Nearly everyone who paid any attention at all to horse racing in the 1970s considers Secretariat to be the greatest racehorse who ever lived. People who never saw him race may wonder how a horse who lost five of his twenty-one lifetime starts at age two and three could be the greatest ever. In 1973, there had not been a Triple Crown winner for 25 years. Many people thought it might never be done again because the three races in five weeks were simply too exhausting for a modern 3-year-old Thoroughbred in May. Then Secretariat exploded with three of the most impressive races in a row. He ran each of the five quarters in the Kentucky Derby faster than his previous quarter mile, setting a new track record. His Preakness was also believed to be a track record but for a suspected timer malfunction. In both races he convincingly defeated outstanding efforts by Sham. In the Belmont Stakes Sham's jockey Laffit Pincay

Jr. pushed Secretariat hard early, but he had to change his strategy mid race. Ron Turcotte on Secretariat continued to fly and finished 31 lengths ahead, breaking the Stakes' record by more than 2 seconds. Pincay actually pulled up Sham short of the finish line.

Secretariat was bred to many of the best broodmares in the world the next 16 years, but he never had a son as spectacular as himself on the racetrack. I remember seeing a very short column in the newspaper announcing that Secretariat was fighting laminitis, and then a day or two later, was a larger column announcing that he had been euthanized due to the "incurable hoof disease." William Nack's report of Secretariat's fight with laminitis was just as brief in his book *Secretariat: The Making of a Champion*. Nack was a racing writer for *Sports Illustrated* who saw Secretariat every day of his two-year racing career. He had very close access to Secretariat's human family and a large part in the movie was based on Nack's book, yet he learned of Secretariat's laminitis and death the next day only because he happened to be in Lexington on other business.

Snowman was the National Champion Open Jumper at Madison Square Garden in the 1950s. He had been purchased off an auction truck on his way to the killers for $80 by Harry DeLeyer. After several years as a school horse at a Long Island boarding school, he was placed in Harry's Jumping string and he went straight to the top. His story is told in a book called *Eighty Dollar Champion*, which was made into a movie. The movie and book mention a very mysterious death. At 25 years old, he wouldn't come out of his stall one morning. The vet returned to euthanize the horse after diagnosing renal failure, but the horse wouldn't leave the stall, just like Dixie, recounted on pages 95-99.

Since I did not see either of these famous horses, I will leave it to the interested reader to find the written accounts and watch the movies for themselves. YouTube carries some paddock video of Secretariat the day before he was euthanized.

# Conclusion

IN ADDITION TO THE SCIENCE and theories of laminitis, this book included over 50 real case histories selected from every variety, cause, and severity of acute laminitis. The cases are taken from Dr. Frederick's actual experience with over 1,200 cases of laminitis in more than 800 real horses and ponies of nearly every breed.

Dr. Frederick only euthanized 26 animals with laminitis from 1974 to 2016. These failures were included, analyzed, understood, and explained so you do not have to repeat them with your horse. None were due to the "mysterious nature of the disease."

Every bad ending was a direct result of our errors in failing to recognize or understand acute laminitis. Most cases are extremely simple, some are very complicated and difficult, but they all have a window of opportunity for correct treatment to prevent crippling founder.

# Principles of Laminitis Treatment

1. Treat the cause, or remove the horse, from the triggering event.
   a. Remove the horse from rich grass. Check the turnout area for toxic plants, especially nightshade, oak, walnut, black cherry, or red maple to see if branches are eaten.
   b. If there has been an acute grain ingestion, give mineral oil orally to speed passage of the grain and prevent acute laminitis.
   c. If the horse has sepsis, retained placenta, or other severe illness, treat it aggressively.
   d. If Cushing's or Equine Metabolic Syndrome is diagnosed, with increased risk of laminitis, discuss this with your vet.
2. Document digital pulses, and check for hoof tenderness, pain on first steps or making a pivot turn in the barn aisle. Flexing a leg for a minute may cause pain in the opposite leg for a few steps when the horse walks off.
3. Give Bute as directed by your vet in doses, adjusting daily, based on the horse's response to ongoing treatment. Diuretics may reduce edema as well.
4. Pull the shoes and trim the toes to facilitate breakover, with squared toes and lowering of the heels.
5. Cool the affected hoofs (cold water preferred rather than ice) and alternate with walking on soft footing.
6. Avoid confining the horse on hard footing.
7. Treatment is likely to be longer if a horse is overweight, is confined on hard footing, has access to leafy hay, grain, or rich pasture, or has had gradual on set and/or delay in diagnosis.
8. Return the horse to work and begin shoeing when off Bute for a minimum of four days with no lameness.
9. Avoid any repeat of the identified triggering events.

# REFERENCES (NOT INCLUDING PAGES 36-42)


1. Frederick D. "Treating Acute Laminitis." *Am. Farriers J.* 1997 Sept-Oct pages 11-18
2. Frederick D. "Laminitis." *J. Eq. Vet. Science* 2003 July;23(7):289
3. Magner D. Magner's *Standard Horse and Stock Book*, 1905:409, 492
4. Obel N. *Studies on the Histopathology of Acute Laminitis.* Uppsala, Sweden: Almquist and Wiskells, 1948
5. Redden R., American Association of Equine Practitioners Convention, Nashville, TN, 1986:747
6. Redden R., American, Association of Equine Practitioners Convention, San Diego, CA. 1988:312
7. Prinz L, McKay-Smith M., "Laminitis." *Equus.* April 1992:174:56-61
8. Pollitt CC, Molyneaux GS. "A Scanning Electron Microscopical Study of the Dermal Microcirculation of the Equine Foot." *Equine Vet. J.* 1990:22(2):79-87
9. Pollitt CC. "Equine Foot Studies Video Tape." School of Vet. Science, University of Queensland, Australia, 1991
10. Garner HE, Coffman Jr, et al. "Clinical Signs of Acute Alimentary Laminitis Correlated with Cardiovascular and Histopathological Alterations." Proceedings 25th American Association of Equine Practitioners Conv. 1974:61-65
11. Hood DM, Grosenbaugh DA, Mostafa MB, et al. "The Role of Vascular Mechanisms in the Development of Acute Equine Laminitis." *J. Vet. Int. Med*, 1993;7:229
12. Coffman JR, Johnson JH, Guffy MM, Finocchio EJ. "Hoof Circulation in Equine Laminitis." *J. Am. Vet. Med. Assn.* 1970:156,76-83
13. Coffman JR, Garner HE. Acute Laminitis. *J Am Vet Med Assn*, 1972:161:1280
14. Garner HE. "Pathophysiology of Equine Laminitis." Proceedings 26th American Association of Equine Practitioners Conv. 1975:21:384-387

15. Hood DM, Amoss MS, Hightower D, et al. "Equine Laminitis I: Radioisotopic Analysis of the Hemodymamics of the Food During the Acute Disease." *J. Equine Med. Surg.* 1978:2:439-444

16. Allen D, Clark ES, Moore JN, Prasse K. "Evaluation of Equine Digital Starling Forces and Hemodynamics During Early Laminitis." *Am. J. Vet. Res.* 1990; 51:1,930-1,934

17. Redden RF. "Hoof wall resection as a treatment in laminitis." In: Proceedings, American Association of Equine Practitioners; 1987. p. 647–56

18. Belknap JK. "Laminitis in Horses." *Merck Veterinary Manual.* Accessed online: https://www.merckvetmanual.com/musculoskeletal-system/lameness-in-horses/laminitis-in-horses

19. Most LO, et al. *Yearbook of Agriculture,* USDA, 1942:456

20. Goetz TF. "The Treatment of Laminitis in Horses." Vet. Clinics of NA 1989:80-82

21. Baxter G. "Current Therapy in Equine Medicine" 3, 1992:157

22. Kobluk CN, Ames TR, Geor RJ. "The Horse," WB Saunders, 1995:676

23. Collins LG, Tyler DE. "Phenylbutazone Toxicosis in the Horse: A Clinical Study." *J. Am. Vet. Med. Assn.*, 1984: 184:669-703

24. Snow DH, Douglas TA, Thompson H, et al. "Phenylbutazone Toxicity in Ponies." *Vet. Rec.* 1979; 105:26-30

25. MacAllister CG. "Effects of Toxic Doses of Phenylbutazone in Ponies." *Am. J. Vet. Res.* 1983; 44:2277-2279

26. MacKay RJ, French TW, Nguyen HT, et al. "Effects of Large Doses of Phenylbutazone Administration in Horses." *Am. J. Vet. Res.* 1983; 44:774-780

27. Weir EK, Lopez-Barneo J, Buckler KJ, Archer SL. "Acute Oxygen-sensing Mechanisms." *N. Engl. J. Med.* 2005 Nov 10;353(19):2042-55. (Comments N. Engl. J. Med. 2006 Mar. 2; 354:9)

28. Hunt RJ. "A Retrospective Evaluation of Laminitis in Horses." *Equine Vet. J.* 1993 Jan.; 25:61-4

29. Donaldson MT, Jorgensen AJ, Beech J. "Evaluation of Suspected Pituitary Pars Intermedia Dysfunction in Horses with Laminitis." *J. Am. Vet Med. Assoc.* 2004 Apr. 1;224(7):1123-7

30. Kane AJ, Traub-Dargatz JL, Losinger WC, et al. "A Cross-Survey of Lameness and Laminitis in U.S. Horses." In Salman MD, Morley PS, Ruch-Gallie R (eds): Proc. 9th Internat. Symp.Vet. Epidem. Econ., Breckenridge, Colorado 2000

31. Frederick D. "Veterinarian's Silence and Excessive Stall Confinement Hurts Laminitis Progress." *Int. Equine Vet.* 2016;6(2):6-11

32. Chapman B, Platt G. Laminitis "American Association of Equine Practitioners Convention," Dallas, TX, 1984:99-109

33. Cited in Coleman MC, Cohen ND. "American Association of Equine Practitioners Foundation Case-Control Study of Pasture-and Endocrinopathy-Associated Laminitis." AAEP Proceedings 2012; 58(3):153-16

34. Frederick D. "Back from the Brink (Fame)." *EQUUS* 2000 June; 272: 35-40

35. Hood D, Stephens KA. "Pathophysiology of Equine Laminitis." *Comp. Cont. Educ. Pract. Vet.*, 1981:3LS454-459

36. Eustace RA, Cripps PJ. "Factors Involved in the Prognosis of Equine Laminitis in the UK." *Equine Veterinary Journal*, 1999;31(5): 433-443

37. Jordan VJ, Ireland JL, Rendle DI. "Does Oral Prednisolone Treatment Increase the Incidence of Acute Laminitis." *Eq. Vet J.* 2016 (29 December); 49(1): 19-25

38. Frederick J., "'Joey'" the Most Severe Acute Laminitis from Fatal Vitamin K3-Kidney Failure." *International Equine Veterinarian* 2016; 6(2): 26-30

39. Rebhun WC, Tennant BC, Dill SG, King JM. "Vitamin K3-induced renal toxicosis in the horse." *J. Am. Vet. Med. Assoc.* 1984 May 15;184(10): 1237-9

40. Cassens DL. "Laminitis Caused by Black Walnut Wood Residues." *Purdue Extension Services Publication* FNR-254 Purdue University, West Lafayette, IN. January 2005

41. USDA-NAHMS "Lameness and laminitis in US horses." Fort Collins, CO. National Animal Health Monitoring System; 2000

# About the Author

*Dr. David Frederick*

HE WAS A COMPETITIVE RACER himself before he ever met a racehorse, or any type of horse for that matter. David Frederick was an excellent high school student and athlete, whose best event was the half-mile run. He was introduced to the horse world during a chance meeting with an airline pilot in his summer job after his first year of college. The pilot owned a state-of-the-art racehorse training farm, and that was an easy connection for a guy whose high school record in the half mile would go unbroken for over 30 years. When Frederick returned to the University of Wisconsin that fall, he switched his major from math to pre-med, which ultimately led to a transfer to the University of Illinois to study veterinary medicine and earn his DVM degree.

Dr. Frederick's always-questioning style of learning continued after veterinary school as he projected his years of "two-legged racing" onto the four-legged patients he encountered as a private practice horse doctor.

From his equine practice in Barrington, Illinois, Dr. Frederick saw countless cases of Laminitis, a crippling condition which can be fatal in severe cases. The lack of consistently successful treatments available during those years led Dr. Frederick on a journey of discovery for his patients and horse owners everywhere.

For 42 years, he did it his way, and made amazing progress saving horses of all types from what others considered an all but unavoidable fate once Laminitis was diagnosed. "That's the way it's always been done," or "It's a mysterious disease, and there really is no cure," did not pass his commonsense style of reasoning. Often in opposition to the consensus derived from pharmaceutically financed or university research-driven clinical trials, Dr. Frederick's own one-at-a-time "clinical trials" on more than 1,200 horses led him to discover and confirm the findings you will read about in the many actual case studies in this book.

Made in USA - Kendallville, IN
13131_9781953294227
02.24.2022 1409